Business Fundamentals

for the *Rehabilitation Professional*

Second Edition

Business Fundamentals

for the Rehabilitation Professional

Second Edition

Tammy Richmond, MS, OTRL
Ultimate Rehab, LLC
Pacific Palisades, California

Dave Powers, PT, DPT, MA, MBA
Ultimate Rehab, LLC
Pacific Palisades, California

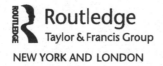
Routledge
Taylor & Francis Group

NEW YORK AND LONDON

First published 2009 by SLACK Incorporated

Published 2024 by Routledge
605 Third Avenue, New York, NY 10158

and by Routledge
4 Park Square, Milton Park, Abingdon, Oxon OX14 4RN

Routledge is an imprint of the Taylor & Francis Group, an informa business

Library of Congress Cataloging-in-Publication Data

Richmond, Tammy.
  Business fundamentals for the rehabilitation professional / Tammy Richmond, Dave Powers. -- 2nd ed.
     p. ; cm.
  Includes bibliographical references and index.
  ISBN 978-1-55642-883-8 (alk. paper)
 1. Medical rehabilitation--Practice. I. Powers, Dave. II. Title.
  [DNLM: 1. Practice Management. 2. Rehabilitation. 3. Professional Practice. WB 320 R533b 2009]
  RM930.R49 2009
  617'.03068--dc22

                                    2008050665

ISBN: 9781556428838 (pbk)
ISBN: 9781003522799 (ebk)

DOI: 10.4324/9781003522799

DEDICATION

In memory of my dear friend and colleague, Linda Botten, OTRL, CHT.

To my beautiful and inspiring daughter, India.

CONTENTS

Chapter 1   **Getting Started** 1
Tammy Richmond, MS, OTRL
  Step 1: Perform Self Assessments and Practice Assessments
  Step 2: Identify Your Business Opportunities
  Step 3: Analyze Your Business Opportunities
  Step 4: Create Vision, Value, and Mission Statements

Chapter 2   **Business Structure** 23
Tammy Richmond, MS, OTRL
  Step 1: Determine Your Tax Status
  Step 2: Determine Your Legal Structure
  Step 3: Create Your Organizational Structure
  Step 4: Select Your Business Name

Chapter 3   **Business Plan** 45
Tammy Richmond, MS, OTRL
  Step 1: Develop Your Business Plan
  Step 2: Secure the Details

Chapter 4   **Marketing Plan** 77
Tammy Richmond, MS, OTRL
  Step 1: Analyze Your Market
  Step 2: Create a Marketing Plan
  Step 3: Implement Your Marketing Plan
  Step 4: Assess and Redirect Your Market Strategies

Chapter 5   **Implementation** 95
Dave Powers, PT, DPT, MA, MBA; Tammy Richmond, MS, OTRL
  Step 1: Gather Advice and Consultation From Experts
  Step 2: Complete Your Operational Infrastructure
  Step 3: Build Your Management Skills and Standards of Care
  Step 4: Promote Professional Competency and Code of Ethics

Chapter 6   **Financial Management** 115
John Richmond, CLU, ChFC; Tammy Richmond, MS, OTRL
  Step 1: Understand Accounting Basics
  Step 2: Manage Your Cash Flow
  Step 3: Improve Your Profitability and Manage Your Risks
  Step 4: Understand the Basics to Billing and Reimbursement

Chapter 7   **Reflect and Redirect** 133
Beverly Sumwalt, MT (ASCP), MA; Tammy Richmond, MS, OTRL
  Step 1: Reflect on Performance and Productivity
  Step 2: Redirect to Enhance Profit and Reduce Expenses

Access to updated and pertinent web addresses containing valuable information about the topics covered in this book can be found at www.routledge.com/9781556428838/

ACKNOWLEDGMENTS

A special thank you to the contributing authors, John Richmond and Beverly Sumwalt.

ABOUT THE AUTHORS

Tammy Richmond, MS, OTRL, is partner of Ultimate Rehab, LLC, Pacific Palisades, CA and an owner of a clinical private practice called Hands 4 Health. She is an adjunct professor at USC, a legal expert, and an author. She also holds positions in state association committees.

Dave Powers, PT, DPT, MA, MBA, is partner of Ultimate Rehab, LLC, Pacific Palisades, CA and an owner of a clinical private practice. He holds positions within the national and state Physical Therapy Associations, holds faculty positions at Mount St. Mary's College, Los Angeles, CA and University of Southern California, Los Angeles, CA, and serves as an expert witness and investigator for the State of California Licensing Board.

CONTRIBUTING AUTHORS

John Richmond, CLU, ChFC, is principle owner of Richmond Financial Services, an independent comprehensive wealth planning and management practice in Milwaukee, WI. He is a current member of the Wisconsin General Agents Hall of Fame, a former member of the Foundation Board of Lutheran Social Services of Wisconsin and Upper Michigan, and past president of the state of Wisconsin's General Agents and Management Association.

Beverly L. Sumwalt, MT (ASCP), MA, is the owner of consulting services in health care clinical operations and e-business. She is also a project team, leadership, and management trainer, writer, and lecturer for the Defense Institute for Medical Operations. She is a member of the Clinical Laboratory Management Association, Medical Group Management Association, American College of Healthcare Executives, and San Diego Organization of Healthcare Leaders, San Diego, CA.

PREFACE

Business Fundamentals for the Rehabilitation Professional, Second Edition is an interactive workbook for rehabilitation professionals and entrepreneurs that answers the "what, where, how, when, and how much" questions of transforming a health care practice idea into a successful business. The workbook is designed to consolidate small business information and tools with health care operations, management, and regulations.

Building upon the first edition, the revised edition takes the reader to the next level of understanding and implementing successful business operations by the introduction to applications of management principles; implementation of evidence-based practice, management, and staff development; expanded coverage of nonprofit business models; and a more in-depth look at reimbursement and financial management. These concepts are woven into the content of the revised book so the reader benefits from the fundamentals of the first book.

Additionally, the revised edition keeps the user-friendly format structure of a workbook and adds additional up-to-date tips and tools for easy reference. Each chapter will continue to ask the reader to apply the content to chapter objectives and questions to assure the understanding and application of the material presented. Worksheets, templates, and tips provide a step-by-step "how-to" approach in taking your business idea and creating an up-and-running successful and compliant health care practice. Access to updated and pertinent web addresses containing valuable information about the topics covered in this book can be found at the following Web address:

www.routledge.com/9781556428838/businessfundamentals

How to Use This Book

This book is filled with lots of exercises, worksheets, and information. Feel free to move around in the book, since starting or expanding a private practice encompasses many business activities at once and not necessarily in a set order. The term "rehab professional" is used to define any health care professional, especially occupational and physical therapists, whose goal is to own and operate his or her own business.

Each chapter builds upon the information of the previous one, but can also act alone to provide you with small business ownership fundamentals and health care practice operations and management. Each chapter contains objectives, summaries, action plans, and a special section for rehabilitation professionals. Words in italics are defined in the glossary. The appendices contain worksheet forms or examples that complement the learning process in the step-by-step workbook format. The information contained in Appendix A may be reproduced for use in connection with your business, but it is not to be given, sold, reproduced, or transmitted in any other form or by any means or use without express written consent of the publisher or authors.

There are 15 basic steps to starting your own health care business:

1. Perform a self-assessment and business assessment.
2. Create a vision statement.
3. Create a mission statement.
4. Define your business concept.
5. Choose your legal structure.
6. Choose your organizational structure.
7. Research and register business names.
8. Write a business plan.
9. Prepare a marketing plan.
10. Obtain advice from experts.
11. Complete start-up tasks.
12. Hire staff.
13. Implement and manage business operations.
14. Manage your finances.
15. File quarterly and annual compliance reports.

The business fundamentals overview algorithm on the next page summarizes the steps involved in establishing a successful health care business.

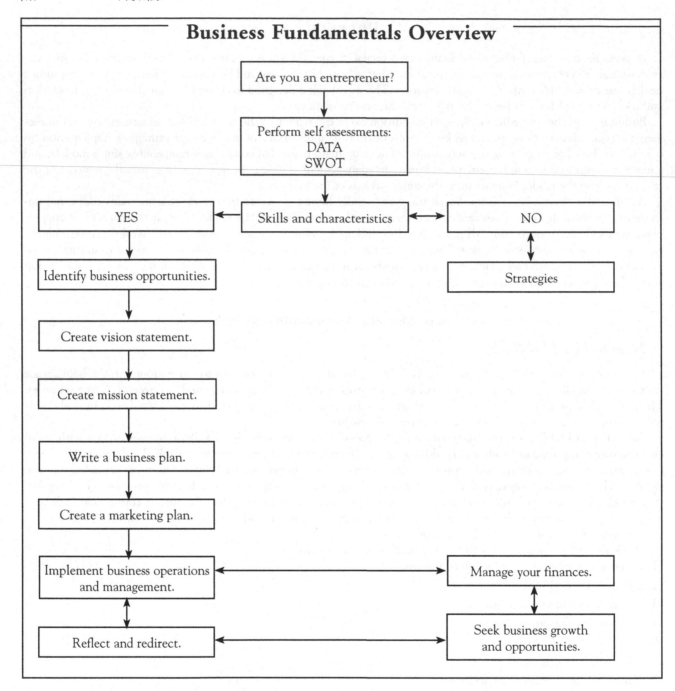

Business Fundamentals Overview

Are you an entrepreneur?

↓

Perform self assessments:
DATA
SWOT

↓

YES ← Skills and characteristics ↔ NO

↓ ↕

Identify business opportunities.　　　Strategies

↓

Create vision statement.

↓

Create mission statement.

↓

Write a business plan.

↓

Create a marketing plan.

↓

Implement business operations and management. ← → Manage your finances.

↕ ↕

Reflect and redirect. ← → Seek business growth and opportunities.

Any successful health care business requires a team of experts to advise, support, and assist in business and health care compliance. The information presented in this book is not to be interpreted as specific legal, accounting, or operational advice for any specific provider. Laws, regulations, and procedures change frequently, and professionals can interpret them differently. For advice on your specific situation, consult an expert. No book or other published material is a substitute for personalized advice from a knowledgeable licensed lawyer, certified accountant, certified or registered financial planner or adviser, or small business or health care consultant.

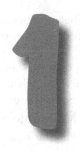

GETTING STARTED

Tammy Richmond, MS, OTRL

CHAPTER OBJECTIVES

✔ Perform self-assessments and practice assessments.
✔ Identify your business opportunities.
✔ Analyze your business opportunities.
✔ Create vision, value, and mission statements.

Health care has become a business model of continuous shifting of health care costs, health care delivery systems, payment mechanisms, and professional responsibilities. Rehabilitation (rehab) professionals are experiencing the transformation of traditional health care work settings into emerging service businesses where knowledge of health care operations and profit-making is a must.

Technology advancements in advanced mass media allow the consumers to be better informed and cost-conscious about their health care choices. They want accessibility, accountability, and quality care for their money. They expect their health care provider to communicate more openly about their services and how they will be implemented and paid for. Likewise, third party payers expect rehab professionals to demonstrate and document their services through clear clinical reasoning and evidence-based criteria.

To succeed in this present health care environment, rehab professionals must not only be skilled clinicians and managers, they must be knowledgeable in small business operations such as tax and legal codes and guidelines, organizational structures, business plans, marketing plans, and reimbursement and financial management. Additionally, rehab professionals must know themselves, their abilities, and their capabilities.

Ask yourself these questions: Do I have an idea or dream that I want to pursue? Do I have the necessary basic skills and characteristics to succeed as a rehab professional and small business owner? Am I an entrepreneur or leader? Can I become a manager and supervisor?

Chapter 1 will assist you in answering these questions. There are four steps to getting started:

Step 1: Perform self-assessments and practice assessments.

Step 2: Identify your business opportunities.

Step 3: Analyze your business opportunities.

Step 4: Create vision, value, and mission statements.

STEP 1: PERFORM SELF-ASSESSMENTS AND PRACTICE ASSESSMENTS

Rehab professionals tell us that they have considered working for themselves but have never truly explored the idea of becoming an entrepreneur or business owner, or they have never committed the entrepreneurial vision to pencil and paper. Moreover, because most rehab professionals do not have a background in business, they do not know exactly where to start. Getting started begins with recognizing the pros and cons of business ownership.

There are advantages to starting your own business that are very appealing. For example:

- Setting your own schedule
- Making more money
- Having a job you love
- Making your own decisions
- Pursuing a dream

Conversely, the disadvantages can seem alienating. For instance:

- Working long hours
- Taking responsibility for successes or failures
- Putting your money at risk
- Lacking job security

Business ownership also requires that you possess certain characteristics of an *entrepreneur*, a *leader*, and a *manager*. Webster's dictionary defines entrepreneur as "a person who organizes and manages a business undertaking, assuming the risk for the sake of the profit."[1] Most rehab professionals easily understand the terms "organize" and "manage," but the terms "risk" and "profit" sound uncomfortable.

Successful entrepreneurs engage in these tasks:

- They seek out new opportunities recognizing emerging trends and service demands.
- They select feasible opportunities based on personal and professional resources and research.
- They implement skills and knowledge, both innate and learned.
- They engage themselves continuously within their support community and professional networks.
- They recognize the need for constant reflection and redirection.

Entrepreneurs are also leaders and managers. Grady defines leaders as individuals that "inspire, direct, guide, and teach others."[2] They possess the ability to create and communicate a bigger picture that encompasses effective and efficient utilization of people power, and innovative and established service models, and they challenge themselves and others to do the job better. They lead with organized management. Managers are individuals who can "increase efficiency, promote stability, assess situations, and select goals."[2] They administer and maintain the bigger picture by implementing structured daily operations and policies and procedures.

Can you see the commonalities between the entrepreneur, leader, and manager? Successful business owners and rehab professionals:

- Possess essential skills in their area of services
- Understand the basic principals of management, marketing, and finance
- Are disciplined and organized; act ethically
- Engage in team building
- Are action-oriented and self-motivating
- Have self-confidence and effective communication skills
- Are planners and good decision makers
- Have passion and perseverance
- Know when and where to seek assistance from experts. They seek out opportunities that will provide services or products that will deliver value and benefits to the client.

In addition, rehab professional entrepreneurs need to be technically skilled and qualified clinicians, be able to adhere to their professional scope of practice and ethical guidelines, be proactive in continuing education in professional and especially business education, and be responsible for delivering and monitoring qualified health care services and products.

✛ Perform Self-Assessments

How do you know if you possess the skills and characteristics of a successful entrepreneur and/or rehab professional business owner? Performing self-assessments will allow you to identify your strengths and weaknesses and assist you in recognizing opportunities for personal growth and entrepreneurial business ideas.

DATA Self-Assessment

Created by William Bridges, DATA stands for desires, abilities, temperament, and assets.[3]

- *Desires* "represent something you would pursue if you knew how to do so," or your personal interests you want to pursue, such as learning to work with challenged children.
- *Abilities* are qualities that are inherent, learned, accomplished, and needed, such as your clinical treatment skills or personal talents.
- *Temperament* can be thought of as personality, attitude, or characteristic traits, such as being energetic or shy.
- *Assets* are those resources and experiences that can be used to your advantage (eg, the fact that you may speak more than one language could be a very important asset for future opportunities).

By identifying your desires, abilities, temperament, and assets, you can determine if you have what it takes to become a rehab professional entrepreneur.

Fill in the DATA Assessment Worksheets on pp. 4–7 and then transfer your circled or highlighted words into the DATA Summary Worksheet on p. 8.

Do you recognize your common traits among the summary columns? Do you have characteristics of a successful entrepreneur, a leader, or a manager? Can you identify your strengths and weaknesses? Do you see some possible opportunities?

✛ Perform a SWOT Analysis

The SWOT Analysis is a common evaluative tool utilized in business and health care for determining the viability of a strategy, plan, or idea. It's very effective for rehab professionals already in a management or supervisory position. It can also be used to evaluate a self-assessment to establish whether you are ready to become a business owner or manager or if you need to expand your skills, experience, or support networks.

SWOT stands for *strengths* (ie, those words that express capabilities or assets), *weaknesses* (ie, those words that describe areas of vulnerability or need for improvement), *opportunities* (ie, those words that promote favorable circumstances for business ideas), and *threats* (ie, those words that signal potential limitations).

To complete the SWOT Analysis, label each of your words in the DATA Summary Worksheet with an S for strengths, W for weaknesses, O for opportunities, or T for threats.

If you are already in a management or supervisory position, complete the SWOT analysis by identifying internal or external factors affecting your present practice operations or expansion ideas. Consider the following factors:

- Customer service
- Quality of services
- Operations and profitability
- Staffing and productivity
- Financial management or reimbursement
- Changes in regulations, both professional and governmental
- Changes in the economic environment
- Competition of other services or programs in general area
- Demands and needs of current clients
- Potentiality of new service or program ideas
- Potentiality of emerging trends

DATA Assessment Worksheet

Desires: List all of your desires, interests, or wishes. Then circle the desires that you would truly pursue (eg, fluent in Spanish, start a Wellness Program, win the lottery).

DATA Assessment Worksheet

Abilities: List all of your skills, qualities, accomplishments, core talents, or tasks you do well. Then circle the ones that come naturally or that others have identified (eg, good at multitasking, easily remember people's names, good computer skills).

DATA Assessment Worksheet

Temperament: Make three copies of this list of personality traits or natural dispositions. Circle the words that best describe you (the goal is to be honest). Give a copy of this list to two people you know and have them circle the words that they feel describe you. Collect all of the lists and highlight those words in common.

Energetic	Patient	Flexible
Flaky	Envious	Monotonic
Attentive	Angry	Listener
Disciplined	Responsible	Proactive
Warm	Boring	Reactionary
Friendly	Humble	Talented
Cold	Talkative	Smart
Cool	Detail oriented	Problem solver
Loud	Team player	Hero
Arrogant	Isolative	Confident
Disorganized	Creative	Interesting
Lazy	Workaholic	Info seeker
Easygoing	Follower	Inappropriate
Humorous	Initiator	Decisive
Spender	Resourceful	Risk taker
Thrifty	Insightful	Conservative
Careless	Depressed	Open minded
Procrastinator	Moody	Anxious
Brilliant	Delightful	Nervous
Abusive	Communicative	Immature
Manipulative	Strong-willed	Refreshing
Diversified	Sad	Powerful
Efficient	Joyful	Jealous
Emotional	Ambitious	Fast thinker
Sensitive	Accountable	Dreamer
Leader	Unaware	Indulgent
Passive	Reflective	Serious
Aggressive	Intuitive	Practical
Productive	Complicated	Critical
Quiet	Victim	Gracious
Positive	Bitter	Committed
Negative	Shy	Expressive
Fearful	Spontaneous	Confusing
Unique	Loyal	Straightforward
Curious	Honest	Fighter
Prideful	Truthful	Frail

Reproduced with permission from Bridges W. *Creating You & Co: Learn to Think Like the CEO of Your Own Career.* New York: Perseus Books; 1997.

DATA Assessment Worksheet

Assets: List all of your experiences, areas of expertise, achievements, and emotional, physical, mental, and spiritual advantages from childhood to present day (eg, worked in a nursing home during college, have a sibling with special needs, assisted parents in their home business). Share this list with another person. Have him or her circle the assets he or she identifies with you.

Reproduced with permission from Bridges W. *Creating You & Co: Learn to Think Like the CEO of Your Own Career.* New York: Perseus Books; 1997.

DATA Summary Worksheet

Desires List circled words	**Abilities** List circled words	**Temperament** List highlighted words	**Assets** List circled words

Fill in the SWOT Analysis Chart below with the categorized words. Some words will fit into one or more categories. Base your decision on your own perceptions.

SWOT Analysis Chart	
Strengths (eg, speak Spanish)	**Weaknesses** (eg, disorganized)
Opportunities (eg, have 2 years of experience in home health)	**Threats** (eg, have no management experience)

Answer these questions.

Do my strengths include discipline, organized, adaptive, responsible, information-seeker, communicative, flexible, resourceful, and leader?

❏ Yes ❏ No

Do my opportunities include desires that are realistic and achievable?

❏ Yes ❏ No

Do my weaknesses and threats outnumber my strengths and opportunities?

❏ Yes ❏ No

Special Considerations for the Rehab Professional

Rehab professionals should also perform a second self-assessment specifically addressing rehab issues. Complete the Rehab Practice Assessment on p. 10.

Rehab Practice Assessment

Key Issues	Yes	No, Need Help	Have Resource
I have vision and mission statements.			
I have several referral sources or networking support.			
I have the knowledge and ability to create proper documentation.			
I have current knowledge in billing/coding.			
I have working knowledge in financial planning and can manage money.			
I have current knowledge in contract negotiations. I am competent in performing evaluations, treatment interventions, and consultations within my scope of practice.			
I have management skills including patient, personnel, and administrative skills.			
I have current knowledge in local and state business, legal, and tax law and requirements.			
I have knowledge in marketing strategies.			
I have knowledge in local, state, and national health care regulations.			

The areas I need to increase my knowledge in or seek expert advice:

_____

_____

_____

The areas that I feel comfortable with:

_____

_____

_____

Adapted from Kovacek P. Self-assessment on practice ownership readiness. Available at: http://www.ptmanager.com/self%20assessment%20on%20readiness%20to%20own%20a%20practice.pdf. Accessed September 27, 2008.

Tips and Tools

If you had difficulty in completing the DATA Assessment Worksheets and SWOT Analysis, develop an action plan to personally or professionally improve your entrepreneurial skills or to gain needed business resources. Consider including the following:

- Attend courses, seminars, and classes.
- Join your local or state professional organizations.
- Meet with consultants, experts, or mentors.
- Find mentors in your area of interests.
- Join networking groups or participate in local, state, and national conferences and meetings.
- Interview and/or visit business owners already engaging in health care business.
- Meet with *Service Corps of Retired Executives (SCORE)* for insight to small business ownership.
- Volunteer in your areas of weaknesses and/or interests.

STEP 2: IDENTIFY YOUR BUSINESS OPPORTUNITIES

Opportunities are combinations of ideas, circumstances, and educational background that can grow into viable businesses.

They often present themselves in several ways:

- Hobbies, interests, or talents
- Work experiences
- Recognition of a needed service or product
- Networking with peers or colleagues
- Education or training
- Being asked to create a new program or expand services

Business opportunities also present themselves through emerging trends (ie, those prevailing tendencies toward certain conditions or situations) or emerging job opportunities influenced by external and internal factors. To recognize emerging practice areas, gather information in four areas:

1. Economic forecasts: statistical information explaining what consumers are spending their money on in personal health or health care and where. Visit www.govspot.com or www.health.gov for statistical information.
2. Consumer wants and needs: what services or products are you, your peers, your family and friends, and your local community spending money and time on (eg, Pilates programs or obesity programs)? Write down the services and products that you notice people in your local community are purchasing.
3. Health care industry: what health care services or products are the federal and state health care laws and governmental agencies spending fiscal money on? More specifically, what practice areas are your state and national associations supporting at the governmental level (eg, driving programs for seniors)? Look at both your specific industry websites (AOTA and APTA), trade magazines, and literature, and at popular culture health and fitness magazines and reading materials for emerging health care trends and identified emerging practice areas.
4. Reimbursement strategies: presently, what new services, programs, and products are being paid for or are not going to be paid for by federal and state funds, third-party payers, and private payers? For example, many managed care organizations are now reimbursing for massage, acupuncture, and other wellness services.

Overall, health care practice emerging trend areas can be divided into two main categories:

1. Business opportunities that meet social needs.
2. Business opportunities that meet specific population needs.

Under each category, four service models, or a combination of these emerging service models, should be considered:

1. Prevention programs
2. Wellness programs
3. Educational programs
4. Niche specialty programs

As a health care practitioner, you have the educational foundation to pursue many different business opportunities that will comply with your standards of practice and offer you potential self-employment and business success. Stop here and write down all of the possible emerging trends in the health care industry, and those in which you are interested and have skills or potential skills.

Emerging trends: _____

_____

Opportunities I'm interested in: _____

_____

Special Considerations for the Rehab Professional

Emerging opportunities for health care professionals are often not found in the traditional work setting nor by utilizing traditional interventions, but rather by incorporating the needs and demands of the consumer within their daily frames of contexts or *communities*.

The following is a list of possibilities:

Psychosocial Needs of Children/Youth:	Afterschool programs with expressive arts, stress management, movement therapy
Home Health:	Home modification, design, accessibility, aging in place
Private Practice:	Ergonomic assessments, low vision, life coaching
Industries/Businesses:	Ergonomics, employee wellness, technology/assistive device development
Community Centers:	Health and wellness educational and support groups
Churches:	Wellness, balance, and health classes
Fitness Centers:	Population- or diagnosis-specific programming and services
Hotels/Resorts:	On-call prevention, wellness, or post rehab programs
Doctors offices:	Private practice, case management, consulting
Malls	Community support groups, life skills classes

Unlike many other types of businesses, health care consists of several professionals often performing similar services. Therefore, skills and experience are the most important elements, followed by knowledge. Spend time and money obtaining additional skills and experience. Put together a list of strategies to improve you or your business opportunity (such as taking classes or courses), and volunteer, interview, or visit present rehab practices in areas of interest for your business ideas.

Certain rehab professional business concepts require post-educational certification or similar specific educational training to satisfy state licensure or certification laws and other practice standards. For example, if your rehab business idea is to start a hand clinic within a commercial industrial work setting, you may be required to show competency or certification in hand therapy services. Contact your state and national practice associations for more information. Keep a portfolio of all of your skill building courses, seminars, or classes to show continual competency in your chosen area of therapy services or products.

Tips and Tools

Additional rehab business opportunities or ideas can be discovered at the following sources:

- Physical and occupational therapy state and national association Web sites, listserv chat groups, articles, conferences, and experts in the field: www.apta.org and www.aota.org
- Professional magazines: www.advanceweb.com
- Networking in your community (ie, chamber of commerce, churches, charities, other professionals)
- Online research: www.bls.gov (Bureau of Labor Statistics); www.hobby.org (Craft and Hobby Association); www.forrester.com (technology and research company)
- Observation of local trends in services, products, ads, and purchases

Become aware of emerging trends by starting a file of ideas from articles, magazines, community activities, charity groups, and conversations with friends, colleagues, and peers. Closely observe and recognize characteristics about your potential consumers and what they value about their health, health care, and wellness.

STEP 3: ANALYZE YOUR BUSINESS OPPURTUNITY

Now that you have identified potential business opportunities in Step 2, it becomes necessary to discover whether the opportunity is actually feasible and viable. There are many reasons why new businesses fail, including:

- Inadequate planning
- Lack of expert support
- Cash flow problems

- Procrastination
- Poor location
- Inability to multitask
- Ineffective or too little marketing
- Poor staffing

Without properly analyzing all of the elements that affect health care businesses, you could be setting yourself up for one or more of the failures mentioned above.

✤ Perform Market Research

Conducting *market research* on your business concept can mean the difference between success and failure. Sometimes it is called a "feasibility study." The objective of completing the market research is to confirm that your business idea is reasonable and achievable before spending any more time and money.

Take the time to thoroughly gather as much specific, accurate, and reliable information as possible to answer the necessary questions about your business idea. A great idea may only be that if you don't have enough resources, consumers, and accessibility to meet the demands of starting and operating a rehab business (see Tips and Tools on p. 16 for research resources).

Fill in the Market Research Worksheet.

Market Research Worksheet

Company Description
- What business idea are you interested in starting? _____
- What are the future trends in your industry? _____
- What are the potential threats in your industry? _____
- Do you have a name for your business? _____
- Who are your consumers? _____
- Can they afford to pay for your services? _____
- Who will potentially refer consumers to your business? _____

Services and Products
- What specific or unique services or products will you provide? _____
- How much will these services and products cost? _____
- Is there a need or demand for your services? _____
- How will the consumer benefit from your services? _____
- Are your services and products readily available? _____
- What equipment and medical supplies will you need? _____
- What are your office supply needs? _____

Location
- How much space do you need for your business? _____
- Do you have a location? _____
- Do you plan to lease, own, or work from home? _____
- Is your space safe and accessible? _____
- Does your space meet local and state regulations, and ADA requirements? _____

Competition
- Who are your competitors? _____
- Where are your competitors located? _____

(continued)

Business Operations
- How do you foresee your business structure? _____
- Do you expect to have employees or independent contractors?_____
- Do you have management experience, or will you need to hire experts?_____
- Do you have the necessary documentation requirements?_____
- Do you understand your standards of practice and ethical guidelines? _____
- Do you understand your professional supervisory requirements? _____

Legal and Tax Considerations
- What federal, state, and local tax laws apply to your business? _____
- What federal health care laws apply to you? _____
- What state licensure laws and regulations apply to your business? _____
- What types of contracts will you need?_____

Insurance
- What insurance coverage will be needed? _____
- Do you have professional liability insurance? _____

Financial and Accounting:
- What is your cash flow? _____
- What financing will you need? _____
- How do you plan to collect money? _____
- What bookkeeping and payroll skills do you need? _____
- Who will file necessary taxes and forms?_____
- How do you plan on being reimbursed for your services?_____
- What are your sources of business income?_____

Sales and Marketing
- How do you plan to market your services? _____

✛ *Analyze Your Market Research Results*

Perform a SWOT Analysis (like the one utilized in Step 1) on your Market Research Worksheet answers. Write down those areas that you can identify as strengths, weaknesses, opportunities, and threats (see next page).

✛ *Refine Your Business Idea*

The SWOT Analysis results should indicate what to do and where to go next. The strengths and opportunities need to outweigh the weaknesses and threats. Typically, successful business ideas need to incorporate at least one of the following:
- Offer something new, better, or unique.
- Provide a service not being met.
- Provide a service to a *target market* that is underserved.
- Offer more services or products in one location.
- Reach and service consumers more efficiently and effectively.
- Contain intact business operations, including finance, management, and marketing.

SWOT Analysis Chart	
Strengths	*Weaknesses*
(eg, location is easily accessible and visible)	(eg, have no sales or marketing experience)
Opportunities	*Threats*
(eg, there is space available to rent that already has equipment)	(eg, don't know if I would be working within my scope of practice guidelines)

To rehab professionals, successful health care businesses also need to incorporate at least the following:

- Satisfy a need or demand for a service or product that you can skillfully deliver.
- Attract, obtain, and keep enough consumers to meet costs and make a profit.
- Obtain several referral sources.
- Find a location with parking and accessibility.
- Follow all state and national standards of practice and ethical guidelines.
- Possess knowledge of where to get expert advice and assistance.

Special Considerations for the Rehab Professional

Failing to thoroughly research and satisfy the elements of a successful health care business may result in financial failure, illegal operations, and professional behavior improprieties. Seek out experts, including private practice owners, consultants, small business experts, lawyers, real estate agents, and financial planners.

There are other rehab professional business concept options to consider. You can buy an existing health care business, partner with other rehab professionals, or contract out your services as an independent contractor or consultant. It may make professional sense, financial sense, and time-saving sense to share or alleviate risks, money, and time. If you decide to buy a practice, hire professional help to obtain a formal appraisal besides your own analysis of the present practice operations, management, consumer base, community, and area market. Partnerships can assist in the work, share in the financial needs and risks, and eliminate sole responsibility, but choosing a partner takes careful consideration and an honest approach. You need to clearly know each other's strengths, weaknesses, and integrity.

Independent contracting and consulting are easier business concepts to start off with because the necessary legal documentation and start-up tasks are simple and uncomplicated, as you will find out in Chapter 2. However, more skill and experience are often necessary to succeed with contracts within independent work environments that offer little input to your services and products. You need good people skills and added flexibility.

Tips and Tools

There are several resources to assist in completing your marketing research worksheet, such as:

- www.bls.gov
- www.bea.gov
- www.insurancenoodle.com
- www.usa.gov
- www.nolo.com

To assist in refining your business concept, visit small business resources such as:

- www.sba.gov
- www.startupbiz.com
- www.gosmallbiz.com
- www.how-to.com

See Appendix I for more resources.

STEP 4: CREATE VISION, VALUE, AND MISSION STATEMENTS

Typically, business or management books teach you these three statement concepts the other way around—mission statement, value statement, and vision statement. However, without a vision, you have no mission. Without values that are inherent in your vision, you have no substantive business goals and sustainability.

Therefore, this book will teach you how to think through the important process of establishing who and what you are logically. You will first develop your vision, then identify your values, and then create the all-important mission statement, which should reflect the first two concepts in obtainable business goals.

David defines vision as "a mental picture of your desired future state filled with vivid 3-D pictures."[4] It answers the creative question, "What do I want my life, including my career, to look like?"

As a rehab professional, the *vision statement* is the mental picture of what you and your health care business concept inspire to contribute and achieve in a global sense, such as advancing preventive care. It motivates you to reach goals. The core motivation of rehab professionals is generally to meet the needs of clients by providing services or products. However, the environment that successfully supports that motivation needs to be imagined and depicted. It needs to be understood by the business owner(s) and the community or market that it serves. By creating a vision statement, the rehab professional or business owner establishes a clear picture of motivational concepts and goals.

✛ Understand the Visioning Process

There are six qualities of a vision statement according to Scott et al[5]:

1. It motivates and inspires.
2. It is a stretch and moves toward greatness.
3. It is clear and concise.
4. It is achievable and not a fantasy.
5. It fits with the highest values.
6. It is easy to communicate, and is clear and simple.

To begin creating a vision statement, first identify your personal goals. Second, determine a bigger picture business idea goal. Sohnen-Moe defines goals as "those things to which you commit and take action to ensure their attainment."[6] Goals should be SMARTER: specific, measurable, attainable, realistic, time-bound, enthusiastic, and rewarding.[6] Like in a clinical setting, you can have short-term and long-term goals.

Complete the statements below:

- What are two personal goals that I would like to achieve (eg, volunteer in the community more often)?
  1. _____
  2. _____
- What is my overall big-picture business goal that I would like to achieve (eg, start my own company)?
  1. _____
- What overall concept or desire do I want my business to address (eg, promote quality of life and proactive choices)?
  1. _____

Vision Statement

Your vision statement is the combination of your desires and goals. Go back to your DATA Summary Worksheet and look at the words under "desires." Can you match some of those desires to your goals indicated above? Attempt to summarize your desires and goals into one concise (25 words or less) paragraph describing what you want your life and career to look like (eg, become a consultant to area businesses promoting work environment adaptation and ergonomics so I can work from home and spend more time with my family; utilize my talents and experience to create a product catalogue of safety devices for homebound clients and sell it; or, establish a sports-specific fitness and injury prevention clinic near area high schools or colleges to promote my skills and community involvement).

Vision Statement: _____

_____

_____

As an example: AOTA's 2017 centennial vision statement reads, "We envision that occupational therapy is a powerful, widely recognized, science-driven, and evidence-based profession with a globally connected and diverse workforce meeting society's occupational needs."[7] The 2020 vision statement for APTA reads, "By 2020, physical therapy will be provided by physical therapists who are doctors of physical therapy, recognized by consumers and other health care professionals as the practitioners of choice to whom consumers have direct access for the diagnosis of, interventions for, and prevention of impairments, functional limitations, and disabilities related to movement, function, and health."[8]

✢ Value Statement

An important fundamental task that can also be included in Step 2 is the development of a *value statement. Values* can be thought of as belief systems, ideals, standards, or codes of ethics. In health care, rehab professionals share a common value of wanting to make people feel better through specific services or interventions. The value statement supports and collaborates the vision statement with actions or behaviors that represent you and your underlying business foundation of commitment and purpose.

Answer these questions:

What do I stand for? _____

What does my work mean to me? _____

How do I want people to view me? _____

How do I want to be treated, and how do I want to treat others? _____

What are my belief systems? _____

What characteristics or behaviors do I value? _____

What is my professional code of ethics? _____

What are my practice standards? _____

How do I want people to view my business? _____

Value Statement:

My purpose or commitment is to: _____

_____

_____

✢ Define Your Purpose

A *mission statement* is a clear, precise statement of the purpose of your business or rehab business idea. It contains the who, what, and how of your business vision and goals. The mission statement serves as an important communication tool and guide for both your business organization and the community in which it will serve. Mission statements are often used on marketing materials and are a must for your *business plan.*

If you are expanding your health care practice into new services or programs, there should already be a mission statement established. Reread the mission statement so that any new services or programs align themselves within the "mission" of the present health care business. Otherwise, you will need to rewrite the mission statement to encompass the broader "what" and uniqueness of the new services or goals.

To create a mission statement, answer the questions below. Keep your selected business ideas from Step 3 in mind.

- Who are you (eg, the name of your business, such as Sunset Home Health Agency or PT Integrated Health Center)?_____

- What are your purpose, goals, services, and/or products (eg, promotes mental health services or advances quality hand therapy services)?_____

  _____

- How are you going to accomplish the goals, services, and/or products (eg, by establishing afterschool programs or by integrating innovative wellness services)?_____

  _____

Mission Statement

Now, summarize the answers into your mission statement (preferably 25 words or less): (eg, "Ultimate Rehab, LLC offers innovative Rehab Practice and Management Consulting services to assist health care providers in establishing a profitable private practice.") _____

_____

_____

As an example: AOTA's mission statement reads, "The American Occupational Therapy Association advances the quality, availability, use, and support of occupational therapy through standard-setting, advocacy, education, and research on behalf of its members and the public."[9] APTA's mission statement reads, "The mission of the American Physical Therapy Association, the principal membership organization representing and promoting the profession of physical therapy, is to further the profession's role in the prevention, diagnosis, and treatment of movement dysfunctions and the enhancement of the physical health and functional abilities of members of the public."[10]

Special Considerations for the Rehab Professional

Mission statements can be confused with a business or company description. Health care companies often print their mission statements on their marketing materials, such as brochures or newsletters. Gather several examples of mission statements, and write down the words that exemplify your objectives and describe your overall services. The goal is to formulate your mission statement to be as precise as possible. The mission statement in rehab management, like the vision statement, is a fundamental documentation tool that is a part of strategic planning. The mission statement provides focus and direction for the organization or business.

CHAPTER 1 SUMMARY

Starting or expanding a successful business requires that you identify four important concepts:

Step 1: Perform Self-Assessments and Practice Assessments

- Are you an entrepreneur? Write down your key personal and business characteristics that exemplify your strengths, weaknesses, opportunities, and threats.

S:_____

W:_____

O: _____

T:_____

Step 2: Identify Your Business Opportunities

- Is your business idea feasible, reasonable, and achievable?   ❐ Yes   ❐ No

Step 3: Analyze Your Business Opportunities

- According to the market research, is your business idea feasible? ❐ Yes   ❐ No

Step 4: Create Your Vision, Value, and Mission Statements

- Write your vision statement.

_____

_____

- Write your value statement.

_____

_____

- Write your mission statement.

_____

_____

Action Plan
    ❐ Continue with the current business concept.
    ❐ Develop personal strategies to achieve the necessary tasks or skills that will make the business concept feasible.

To prepare yourself for becoming a business owner, take the time to research and learn how to perform the necessary skills indicated, or be able to hire experts to perform or advise you on the various areas of your weaknesses or threats.

Recognizing now that you are not able or willing to work the long hours and take the risks involved in business ownership will save you from potential failure. Not all people are meant to be entrepreneurs.

REFERENCES

1. *Websters' Dictionary*. 3rd college ed. New York, NY: Simon & Schuster, Inc; 1998:454.

2. Grady D. From management to leadership. In: McCormack G, Jaffe E, Goodman-Lavey M, eds. *The Occupational Therapy Manager*. 4th ed. AOTA Press; 2003:333-345.

3. Bridges W. *Creating You & Co: Learn to Think Like the CEO of Your Own Career*. New York, NY: Perseus Books; 1997.

4. David M. *The Self-Manager Success Journal*. San Mateo, CA: The Mark David Corporation; 2001:8.

5. Scott C, Jaffe D, Tobe G. *Organizational Vision, Values, and Mission*. Menlo Park, CA: Crisp Publications, Inc; 1993:82.

6. Sohnen-Moe CM. *Business Mastery: A Guide for Creating a Fulfilling, Thriving Business and Keeping it Successful*. 3rd ed. Tucson, AZ: Sohnen-Moe Associates, Inc; 1988.

7. HighBeam Research. AJOT and AOTA centennial vision. Available at: http://www.highbeam.com/doc/1P3-1281732971.html. Accessed October 29, 2008.

8. American Physical Therapy Association. APTA vision statement. Available at: http://www.apta.org/vision2020. Accessed October 29, 2008.

9. American Occupational Therapy Association. About AOTA. Available at: http://www.aota.org/general/about.asp. Accessed April 13, 2004.

10. American Physical Therapy Association. APTA mission statement. Available at: http://www.apta.org/AM/Template. cfm?Section=About_APTA&TEMPLATE=/CM/ContentDisplay.cfm&CONTENTID=19077. Accessed December 30, 2008.

SUGGESTED READING

AllBusiness. Do you have the right stuff to be an entrepreneur? Available at: http://www.allbusiness.com/human-resources/careers-changing-jobs/1540-1.html. Accessed October 29, 2008.

American Occupational Therapy Association. Top 10 emerging practice areas to watch in the new millennium. Available at: http://www.aota.org/Practitioners/PracticeAreas/Emerging/36247.aspx. Accessed October 29, 2008.

Baider L. Using mission and vision statements. *Advance for Occupational Therapy Practitioners* [serial online]. 2002;18(11):7. Available at: http://occupational-therapy.advanceweb.com/Editorial/Search/AViewer.aspx?AN=OT_02jun3_otp7.html&AD=06-03-2002. Accessed October 29, 2008.

Behar E. Blueprint for success: thinking about starting a private practice? Review these basics. *Advance for Directors in Rehabilitation*. 2002;11(8):15-16.

Brown EJ. Why private practice insurance is not the answer to the mandate dilemma. *Advance for Occupational Therapist Practitioners* [serial online]. 2008;24(5):16. Available at: http://occupational-therapy.advanceweb.com/Editorial/Search/AViewer.aspx?AN=OT_08mar3_otp16.html&AD=03-03-2008. Accessed October 29, 2008.

Diamond L. Carving out a niche. Available at: www.rehabpub.com/rehabec/12002/2.asp. Accessed November 4, 2008.

Diffendal J. Profiles in private practice. *Advance for Occupational Therapy Practitioners* [serial online]. 2001;17(25):12. Available at: http://occupational-therapy.advanceweb.com/Editorial/Search/AViewer.aspx?AN=OT_01dec10_otp12.html&AD=12-10-2001. Accessed October 29, 2008.

Fahey L, Randall RM. *The Portable MBA in Strategy*. New York, NY: Wiley; 1994.

Handle D. How-to create a mission statement. Available at: http://www.how-to.com/article/details/105/how-to-create-a-mission-statement.html. Accessed December 30, 2008.

Kovacek P. Practice ownership success readiness. Available at: http://www.ptmanager.com/self%20assessment%20on%20readiness%20to%20own%20a%20practice.pdf. Accessed September 27, 2002.

Kovacek P. Ready to be an entrepreneur? *Advance for Physical Therapists and PT Assistants* [serial online]. 2002;13(16):17. Available at: http://physical-therapy.advanceweb.com/Editorial/Search/AViewer.aspx?AN=PT_02aug5_ptp7.html&AD=08-05-2002. Accessed October 29, 2008.

Nosse L, Friberg D, Kovacek P. *Managerial and Supervisory Principles for Physical Therapists*. Philadelphia, PA: Williams & Wilkens; 1999.

Pinson L, Jinnett J. *Steps to Small Business Start-Up*. 4th ed. Chicago, IL: Dearborn; 2000.

Steib P. Going solo: is it the right move for you? Available at: http://www.otjoblink.org/links/link13.asp. Accessed April 21, 2002.

Strickland R. Strategic planning. In: McCormack G, Jaffe E, Goodman-Lavey M, eds. *The Occupational Therapy Manager*. Bethesda, MD: American Occupational Therapy Association, Inc; 1996:51-63.

Thrash J. The hidden treasures of an OT career. *Advance for Occupational Therapists* [serial online]. 2008;24(3):14. Available at: http://occupational-therapy.advanceweb.com/Editorial/Search/AViewer.aspx?AN=OT_08feb4_otp14.html&AD=02-04-2008. Accessed October 29, 2008.

Tinsley R. On your own: if you're a new practice owner, follow these basic rules. *Advance for Directors in Rehabilitation* [serial online]. 2001;10(8):13. Available at: http://rehabilitation-director.advanceweb.com/Editorial/Search/AViewer.aspx?AN=DR_01aug1_drp13.html&AD=08-01-2001. Accessed October 29, 2008.

Weinper M. Private practice premonitions, the sequel. *Rehab Management.* 2004;17(1):48-57.

ELECTRONIC RESOURCES

www.entrepreneurship.com: Online site to global entrepreneurship with education, research, and events.

www.federalnewsradio.com: Online and AM radio station with the latest federal government news.

www.toolkit.com: Online business owners' resource for small business operations and templates.

BUSINESS STRUCTURE

Tammy Richmond, MS, OTRL

In business operations, the term *business structure* is often used synonymously with the term *legal structure*. For our purposes, business structure is the organizational outcome of several business tasks that legally defines a business entity. The business concept that you identified in Chapter 1 now needs to be defined by tax, legal, and organizational parameters in order to comply with federal, state, and local business and health care laws. Your business structure will be the legal structure under which you conduct your rehab business operations. These important business principles will become part of your business plan and ultimately decide the direction of implementing your rehab business concept.

There are four steps to advancing the development of your business concept into a viable rehab health care business structure. They are:

Step 1: Determine your tax status.
Step 2: Determine your legal structure.
Step 3: Create your organizational structure.
Step 4: Select your business name.

Business structures generally differ by size, ownership, control, tax, and liability (risks) considerations. The type of final business structure you choose is based on your unique, personal, and rehab business objectives, and the legal and tax opportunities or limitations available by federal, state, and local laws and regulations. Obtain expert assistance from an attorney, tax accountant, or a local small business consultant since many federal, state, and local tax and business laws change frequently and are subject to situational considerations. For example, in California, occupational therapists cannot form a limited liability company (LLC) and hire physical therapists or speech pathologists. However, the three disciplines could form a corporation and, therefore, satisfy both small business and health care laws and regulations.

Gathering and acquiring accurate and reliable information in determining your business structure, including health care regulations, can be time-consuming and frustrating. Even experts can differ on which business structure is best for your rehab business concept. Federal and state health care regulations may sometimes be interpreted differently between agencies, national organizational bodies, state regulatory boards, consultants, and attorneys. Keep these recommendations in mind:

- Gather as much information as possible from credible sources.
- Make business decisions based on expert opinion and documentation.
- Support your business structure choice and health care operations by identifying and documenting the resources utilized in making your decisions.
- Do not risk your rehab business by foregoing the extra time or money necessary in properly establishing your business structure.
- Ask your state licensing, registration, certification board, or state governing agency if there are regulations or written practice act position papers regarding business structures or business ownership.
- Be sure to read and understand insurance carriers' contracts or other funding entities' credentialing requirements and contracts to be certain that you are meeting their legal structure qualifications.
- Join your national organization, such as APTA and AOTA, and state physical and occupational therapy associations to take advantage of the credible resources and expert advice available.

STEP 1: DETERMINE YOUR TAX STATUS

One of the main objectives of any business is to make a profit from the services or products you provide. Profit can be money, altruism, or both. Regardless, global financial infrastructure is based on a medium of exchange with a measurement of value. You will need money to start, implement, and continue to grow your rehab business concept. A part of your profits will be assessed for taxation.

✚ Understand the Main Types of Business Taxes

The term *tax* is very familiar to us. This is a percentage of money owed to support the federal, state, and local governments.

There are four main general kinds of business taxes that are related to understanding business structures:

1. *Income tax:* Taxes paid on monies or profits made.
2. *Self-employment tax:* Social security and Medicare tax paid by individuals who work for themselves or in a partnership that acts like the withheld employee taxes by employers.
3. *Employment tax:* Federal income tax withholding, social security and Medicare taxes (FICA), and Federal Unemployment Tax (FUTA).
4. *Sales and use tax:* Tax applied to most sale items. Generally, the State Board of Equalization (BOE) governs sales and use tax. If you sell a product, you will have to apply for a seller's permit from BOE and pay quarterly taxes on the taxes that you collected on the products that you sold.

If you are a self-employed rehab professional, you will pay income taxes, self-employment taxes, and, if you sell products, you will also pay sales and use tax. If you work for your own rehab corporation, generally speaking, you will pay income taxes, employment taxes, and sales and use tax, if applicable. Conversely, when you are an employee, monies are taken from your paycheck and directed into Social Security, Medicare, and other federal taxes by your employer.

✚ Identify the Two Main Tax Statuses

A basic first question to ask yourself is, "Is my business structure goal to provide services and products to make profits for myself, or is it to provide services and products with profits?" There are two tax statuses to choose from:

1. *For-profit:* Providing services and products for the purpose of making money for owners.[1]
2. *Nonprofit:* Providing educational or charitable services and products for selected individuals or populations with funded or donated monies.

The most common answer is that you want to make a profit for yourself; therefore, you are a for-profit tax structure. You then need to select a legal structure, pay appropriate required fees and taxes, and operate under certain business and health care laws and regulations.

Nonprofit tax structures are considered tax-exempt (ie, they do not pay federal taxes). However, nonprofit tax structures do have to apply and follow the exemption requirements of the Internal Revenue Service (IRS). Go to www.irs.gov/charities/index.html to read about specific qualifications and procedures. Your state government will also require you to apply for exemption of state income taxes. The services or products you provide will be "volunteered" or "donated," although reasonable compensation for owners is allowed. Excess revenue is required to be reinvested into the nonprofit business to further its mission and vision objectives. The IRS also requires the nonprofit organization to be established as one of four legal structures: a corporation, community chest, fund, or foundation. If you have employees, you may be subject to paying other payroll taxes and other sales and use tax. Obtain further details from the IRS, your state franchise tax board, and the BOE. Seek additional assistance from an accountant, attorney, or small business consultant.

Special Considerations for the Rehab Professional

To better understand how business structure tasks such as tax status and legal structure impact our practice domain in health care, we need to review our various guidelines, policies, and regulations already established by the national and state professional associations; the state government, including state licensing, registration, and certification; and the federal government.

National Associations

The AOTA and APTA are voluntary membership organizations and do not regulate any type of small business tax and legal functions. They do offer official, written documentation and guidelines to standards of practice, codes of ethics, and supervision and delivery of therapy services. If you are a member, you are obligated to abide by the code of ethics and adhere to the standards of practice. AOTA and APTA also provide up-to-date information regarding federal affairs and their impact on professional standards, regulations, and emerging opportunities.

State Associations

Likewise, the state occupational therapy and physical therapy associations are voluntary membership organizations and do not regulate any type of tax and legal business activities. The state associations work in conjunction with the national associations to promote the standards of practice and ethical practice behavior, along with supporting the profession and its members by offering practice and educational information through materials, conferences, seminars, and experts. They also play an important role in promoting the professions to the public and private sectors. In most cases, the state association interacts with the state government in specific industry regulatory issues.

State Government

Practice laws and regulations that occupational and physical therapists and occupational and physical therapy assistants do have to follow are established at the state government level. There are four main types of regulatory laws. They include licensure, mandatory certification, mandatory registration, and trademark law. Typical components of regulations include the definitions of practice and practice issues, educational requirements, supervisory requirements, and disciplinary actions and recourse. Which type of professional regulatory law applies to you is state specific. It is your responsibility to contact your state board or state government to obtain copies of the laws and regulations. You will need to comply with all laws and regulations set forth by the state government, state board, or advisory committee. The national association websites (www.aota.org and www.apta.org) contain the state-by-state regulatory information, or you can contact your state regulatory body directly.

Federal Government

Federal health laws apply to rehab professionals both as federal health care regulations and policies such as HIPAA (Health Insurance Portability and Accountability Act), and government-funded health care programs such as Medicare or Medicaid. Protecting the public by preserving public health is the main objective of federal and state health care laws. Federal health care activities are delegated mainly to the Department of Health and Human Services (HHS; www.hhs.gov) under the Office of Secretary of State. HHS provides more than 300 programs under 11 operating divisions—eight agencies under public health service operations that include National Institutes of Health (NIH) and Centers for Disease Control and Prevention (CDC), and three human services divisions that include Centers for Medicare and Medicaid Services (CMS; www.cms.gov) and Administration on Aging (AoA). Many HHS-funded services are administered through state and local agencies. HHS also provides federal grant programs. If you are going to receive reimbursement either from a state- or federal-funded program, you are required to apply and fulfill all of the requirements and regulatory standards specific to that agency. For example, if your rehab business concept is an early intervention developmental play program for developmentally delayed infants, payment for such services may fall under a federally funded program administered through the corresponding state agency. You may be required to apply to the state agency and follow specific documentation and reimbursement policies and standards

Tips and Tools

A nonprofit organization is a legal entity whose objective is to support or engage in activities of public benefit, often without any commercial or monetary profit. The most common types of nonprofit organization for health care providers are Internal Revenue Code Section 501(c)(3) "public charities." They receive their financial support from the public in the form of grants and private donations. The primary purpose of a nonprofit is to do good things without the purpose of making financial profits. The advantages of forming a nonprofit include: tax exemption, tax deductions for your donors, grant eligibility, public goodwill, and establishing a permanent entity for a social service.

The Internal Revenue Service has established rules of engagement and require an application and both federal and state administrative paperwork that must be followed carefully. The steps to forming a nonprofit organization are quite similar to the steps in forming a corporation. During the tax exemption application process, you are essentially required to create a business plan. Funding sources and/or state law may also require you to obtain an annual audit.

Some helpful websites include:

- Guidestar: www.guidestar.gov
- National Council of Nonprofits: www.councilofnonprofits.org
- Internal Revenue Service: www.irs.gov/charities
- Grant opportunities: www.grants.gov

Adapted with permission from a lecture, "Nonprofit Organizations Primer," by Michael Cantrill, RBZ, LLP given March 25, 2008.

STEP 2: DETERMINE YOUR LEGAL STRUCTURE

The information provided in this step is intended to give you a general understanding of the main types of legal structures and is not to be interpreted as specific legal advice. Legal structures are governed by business law and, therefore, may vary in specific rules and regulations from state to state. You will be required to select one of the four types of legal structures for your business concept to comply with federal, state, and local business and health care laws. Obtaining expert business advice and services from a small business tax expert, accountant, or attorney is highly recommended.

The enforcement of business and health care law regulations can fall under several different governing agencies. Generally speaking, the state governing body enforces the laws and regulations that are state created, and the federal government will enforce the laws that are created by federal government. Each type of organization will internally enforce additional obligations by membership or contract into associations, agencies, networks, and other types of specialty business or health care services organizations.

✦ Explore the Four Types of Legal Structures

Determining your legal structure is your first important legal decision, and it requires gathering some extra information and expert advice. Legal structures are the organizational formations of specific legal business tasks and documentation that define elements of ownership or the relationship between owners, types of businesses, and business objectives, management, and legal operations. They differ from each other by the number of owners or stockholders, liability and risk levels, tax requirements, and ownership control, and they vary in legal complexity. Individual state governments regulate the four types of legal structures. However, all four types may not be available to rehab professionals because of specific governmental regulations. After becoming familiar with the different types of legal structures, you will need to research which types are applicable and available to you and your particular rehab business concept in your state.

There are four general types of legal structures:
1. Sole proprietorship
2. Partnership
3. Corporation
4. Limited liability company (LLC)

Sole Proprietorship

A *sole proprietorship* is the most common and easiest type of start-up business structure. A sole proprietorship is owned and operated by one person, can have employees, and has not filed documents to become a corporation or an LLC. You automatically assume a sole proprietorship legal structure by default if performing work without an employee status and as self-employed, such as a private practice owner, independent contractor, or consultant, regardless if you register a company name. Simply, once you are making money for services rendered and making your own business decisions, even a few hours away from a full-time job or on the side as a hobby, you are a sole proprietorship.

The advantages of a sole proprietorship are as follows:
*   It is easy to form.
*   The owner has complete control.
*   The owner receives all income.
*   There are fewer recordkeeping activities.
*   You can deduct certain itemized business expenses.
*   You pay personal income taxes on business profits and not as a company (ie, "pass-through" taxation).
*   It is easy to dissolve.

The disadvantages of a sole proprietorship include:
*   The owner has all legal and operational responsibilities.
*   The owner is exposed to unlimited personal liability risks.
*   There are limited growth opportunities.
*   Funding usually comes from a sole owner or limited other resources.
*   Some employee benefits, such as your wages, are not directly deductible from business income.
*   It dissolves upon death or impairment to perform business activities.

Here are some of the typical business tasks and forms that are required:
*   Register your fictitious business name or "Doing Business As" (DBA) name with the County Clerk Registrar Recorder Office in the county where your business will be located. This may not be applicable if you are using your name or part of your name as the title of the company. This process also requires that you advertise your fictitious business name out to the public for a period of time to avoid copyright or trademark infringement.
*   Obtain a local tax registration certificate through your local city administration office or county clerk's office. (Sometimes referred to as a business license.)
*   Obtain a seller's permit, or resale number, from your state's BOE if you are selling products. Generally, you are required to pay quarterly sales tax on the sales tax collected by sales of products. Consult with an accountant for more details, or contact your state BOE by typing "Board of Equalization, (name of your state)" in an online search engine (eg, Board of Equalization, California).
*   Obtain specialized licenses or permits such as certificate of occupancy, zoning, fire and building safety, and health inspection. Check with your local city and county administration offices such as the business license office, small business administration (SBA) office, or chamber of commerce.
*   Pay annual federal and state income taxes.
*   Pay estimated quarterly taxes.
*   Pay self-employment taxes.
*   Pay employee tax, if applicable.

- Obtain a *federal employee identification number (EIN)* at www.irs.gov. If there are no employees, you may use your social security number as your tax identification number unless otherwise required by federal law.
- If you have employees, you will need workers' compensation insurance and need to withhold taxes for state disability insurance, personal income tax, and unemployment insurance. Check with the state's employment development department or tax accountant.
- Open a separate bank account for your business.
- Obtain or renew current professional license, registration, or certification requirements through your state licensing board or state government.
- Apply to Medicare for a personal identification number (PIN) for Medicare coverage at www.cms.gov.
- Establish service contracts with third-party payers.

If your rehab business has only one owner, such as working as a consultant, independent contractor, or private practice owner, establishing your legal structure as a sole proprietorship is the simplest option. Most rehab professional business owners start as sole proprietorships because it is the easiest, most flexible, and the least time-consuming legal structure. It is also the least protective against personal risks and business liabilities. If someone were to bring a lawsuit against your sole proprietorship rehab business, your personal assets are vulnerable. It is important to obtain professional liability insurance for liability protection and to be comfortable with the risks. Having written contracts also acts as a legal safeguard and is highly recommended.

Partnership

A *partnership* is a legal business relationship with two or more owners (partners), with or without employees, that has not filed documents as a corporation or an LLC. There is no limit on the type or number of partners (eg, between a rehab professional [individual] and a clinic or another existing therapy partnership group). General partners are those individuals who control the daily operations and share liability. Limited partners usually only contribute financially to a partnership and have minimal input into business operations. The partners share ownership, profits, and losses, but assume separate responsibility for their own professional practice operations and management. However, there are legal risks. In certain types of partnerships, each partner can be held personally responsible for debts and legal obligations of the other partners. For example, if a general partner commits fraudulent medical billing without your knowledge, the partnership, including the other innocent partners, can be held liable. For that reason, a partnership agreement is very important, although not required.

In the absence of a written agreement, your state may engage the Uniform Partnership Act as the standard legal documentation. The default agreement will dictate the terms of the partnership, regardless of how you are operating. Therefore, it is wiser to spend the extra time and money to have a written agreement drawn up by an attorney to address time and money contribution, income payment, decision making, management, and other business operations that is agreeable between all the partners involved.

There are three types of partnerships:
1. General partnerships
   o General partners are personally liable for business operations and debts.
2. *Limited partnerships* or limited liability partnerships
   o They require one general partner and one limited partner.
   o The general partner controls daily operations and is liable for debts.
   o The limited partner has minimal control, no liability, and typically contributes financially.
   o They may be restricted by state law for professional businesses.
3. Joint ventures
   o They are like a general partnership, but only for a limited period of time or for a single project.

Check with a local attorney, tax accountant, or the office of the Secretary of State to determine what types of partnerships are available to your rehab business in the state in which the business will be located.

The advantages of partnerships are as follows:
- They are relatively easy to establish and can have less taxation than corporations.
- There is more working *capital* (money) available.
- Profits/losses from the business may go directly to the partners' personal income tax returns.

- There is a built-in incentive for attracting employees, such as career ladder growth.
- There are shared business operation responsibilities.
- There are increased growth strategies, such as adding partners.

Disadvantages of partnerships include:
- Profits are shared with partners.
- Partners are individually and jointly liable for each other's actions.
- Disagreements between partners can harm business.
- Some employees' benefits are not deductible from business income.
- Partnership may end upon the withdrawal or death of a partner.

Typical business tasks and forms required are:
- All of the same tasks and forms as a sole proprietorship mentioned previously
- A partnership tax return
- A certificate of limited partnership, if applicable
- A written partnership agreement. Basic written partnership agreement forms can often be found and purchased online or through the Secretary of State office and Web site. There is a fee for the agreement form and filing fees. Recommend seeking additional legal or small business consultant assistance.

Rehab professionals should consider a partnership when under these circumstances:
- There is more than one rehab professional owner, such as a group practice.
- You personally know and trust the other rehab professional owners involved.
- You need a financial partner and not just a business loan.
- You have additional insurance protection, such as professional liability insurance.
- A particular job opportunity for a specific purpose and amount of time is best handled as a joint venture or business project with separate business entities working together but operating alone. An example could be a wellness outpatient clinic that is made up of an occupational and physical therapist, an acupuncturist, massage therapist, Feldenkrais practitioner, and a nutritionist. They all form a partnership that shares office space, overhead expenses, and office assistants, but each is in charge of his or her own practice operations and management.

Corporation

A *corporation* is the most complex type of business structure because it legally acts as a completely separate entity from the owner(s) and imposes certain legal and tax rules on its owners, now called "shareholders" or "stockholders." Corporations can have one or more owners or stockholders. Stockholders own stock, which is the total percentage of ownership divided into equal amounts or shares. The person(s) with the largest ownership of stock has more control.

The stockholders are not personally responsible for any losses. For example, if someone filed a lawsuit against one of the owners or employees, the corporation (and not the individuals) would be liable, with a few exceptions. Therefore, your personal assets are generally protected. The stockholders elect a board of directors who manage or supervise the company's operations. The board of directors may appoint officers such as a president or vice president.

There are three common types of corporations: C corporation (or general corporation), subchapter S corporation, and professional corporation or *professional service corporation* (PSC). (The term "association" may also be used and is generally considered a "non-stock" corporation usually used for nonprofit organizations or community associations. Check with an attorney or accountant.)

Each state requires all corporation types to file formal corporate documents and pay initial and annual fees apart from the various federal and state income taxes. Once you file as a corporation, you are considered "incorporated" (Inc). You will also be required to establish bylaws or rules and procedures that must be followed, such as stockholder meetings and a description of officers' responsibilities. This increased amount of documentation is what makes the corporation legal structure a more complicated and time-consuming business structure form. However, the protection of personal assets from losses and lawsuits often outweighs the extensive paperwork.

The advantages of a corporation include:
- Shareholders have limited liability for corporation's debt or lawsuits; therefore, it offers more personal protection.
- Ownership can be easily transferred to another person or entity.
- There are increased options for growth and finances, such as stock options or stock sales.
- Authority can be delegated.
- A deduction of benefit costs is allowed for officers and employees.

The disadvantages include:
- There are extensive governmental regulations and monitoring.
- There are extensive documentation requirements and maintenance.
- They are usually more expensive and time-consuming to formulate.
- Compliance with variable federal laws with interstate business commerce is required if owning a rehab business with companies in more than one state.
- Activities can be limited by state laws.
- The company is capitalized.

The subchapter S corporation differs from the C corporation mainly by taxation. The shareholders in a subchapter S corporation do not pay federal income tax on company profits. Instead, the profits or losses pass directly to the owners' personal income tax and are taxed at individual rates. Accountants may recommend a subchapter S corporation legal structure to rehab professionals because it offers the best protection from personal liabilities and may allow for additional business deductions that the other legal structures do not.

A PSC is a general corporation that can only be owned and operated by licensed professionals. It must meet the requirement that the principal activity of the PSC is the performance of personal services, such as health, law, and accounting. Group practices often choose this legal structure when prohibited from forming an LLC. Each state government decides which professions are allowed to incorporate as PSCs. Therefore, it is important to check with your state regulatory board or agency and an attorney to learn the availability and limitations of this type of legal structure.

Typical business tasks and forms required include:
- All of the tasks and forms mentioned previously under sole proprietorship
- Articles of Incorporation filed with your Secretary of State. The Articles of Incorporation will act as the contract between the stockholders.
- Forms for capital gains, sale of assets, alternative minimum tax, and several other items (assistance is recommended)

Limited Liability Company

An *LLC* is a newer type of legal structure now permissible in most states. It allows owners the personal liability protection of a corporation and the pass-through taxation and operational flexibility of a partnership or sole proprietorship. The owners are commonly called "members," and in some states, a single person may form an LLC and have employees. LLCs are limited to two of the four business characteristics of corporations: continuity of existence, limited liability to the extent of assets, centralized management, and free transferability of ownership interests. An LLC can be taxed as a sole proprietorship, partnership, or corporation.

Certain states will not allow professional services such as physical and occupational therapy to establish their business structure as an LLC. Make sure to check with an accountant, attorney, or other small business expert and the state licensing board for specific state LLC restrictions. If there is more than one owner or member, it is recommended that you establish a written agreement in addition to filing the Articles of Organization. The written agreement contains similar operating and management elements as in a partnership agreement.

The advantages of an LLC include:
- It is easier than forming a corporation.
- There are fewer restrictions on the type and number of owners.
- There are fewer recordkeeping and corporate meeting rules.
- Owners do not assume personal liability for business debt.

- Losses can be used as tax deduction against active income.
- There is flexibility in the allocation of profits and losses versus ownership share.
- There is pass-through taxation to personal tax returns.
- Ownership opportunities are easier.

The disadvantages include:
- Some states impose a corporate tax.
- Some states restrict use with certain professional services, such as physical or occupational therapy.
- There are some restrictions on transferring ownership.
- There is a lack of uniform provisions from state to state.
- There is limited personal protection in some areas.
- The company is capitalized.

Typical business forms required include:
- Articles of Organization filed with your Secretary of State
- All of the tasks and forms mentioned previously under sole proprietorship

Table 2-1 provides you with an overview of the general types of legal structures. Contact your state licensing board to obtain any professional practice regulations regarding legal structures. Attain legal counsel for specific legal advice and services.

Special Considerations for the Rehab Professional

Legal structures and operations may be affected by your state's health care laws and professional regulations. This is where confusion and frustration can arise and professional assistance is absolutely necessary. Keep in mind that even if the state's business laws and regulations allow you, the therapist, to become a rehab business owner, your state licensing, registration, or certification board or governing agency may not. Health care laws and professional regulations will prevail. These two separate but synergistic governing bodies—federal and state business laws and federal and state health care laws—require careful attention to details.

An additional matter to consider in the legal structure selection is adhering to professional practice supervisory requirements and their relationship to business ownership. Review your state's practice supervisory regulations or guidelines. Thoroughly understand the responsibility and work task parameters of assistants, students, limited permit holders, and aides. Occupational and physical therapy assistants may not be able to own their own rehab business because the state therapy board or governing agency prohibits it. Or, the therapy assistant may be able to own and manage but not clinically work or make decisions in the rehab business because of supervisory requirements and regulations.

Furthermore, some state therapy laws and regulations prohibit non-licensed laypersons to own or partner in a health care business. However, they may allow the layperson to take the position of limited partner (financial partner). For example, in the state of California, the physical therapy board published a statement regarding a physical therapy assistant's corporation ownership and physical therapy ownership by laypersons that sets forth specific legal structure provisions.[2] Also, provider networks (see Tips and Tools on p. 33) may restrict ownership to licensed personnel.

Follow these guidelines to assist in determining which legal structure(s) are available in your state and will comply with your state's practice laws and regulations:
- Contact an accountant, small business consultant, or the department of the Secretary of State for legal structure types available to health care professionals. Make sure to specify for-profit or nonprofit, as well as any specific services such as consulting versus clinical services.
- Contact your state therapy licensing board or oversight agency for any documentation regarding business or legal structure practice issues and limitations of ownership. Make sure to specify licensed or certified therapist or therapy assistant, or limited permit holder.
- Spend the additional time or money to meet with a health care lawyer to receive proper legal interpretations, advice, and conclusions. The lawyer may offer several options that are agreeable to satisfy both health care laws and business laws.
- As a general rule of thumb, maintain all documentation to support your final legal structure decision. Laws and regulations can change over time and require annual review.

TABLE 2-1
Comparison of Legal Structures

Things To Consider	Sole Proprietorship	Partnership	Corporation (PSC)	S Corporation	Limited Liability Company	Nonprofit
Number of owners	One individual; Easiest to formulate	Two or more	Unlimited; Some states have a minimum of two	One to 75; Limited types of owners	One or more; State specific	Generally the same as a corporation
Amount of Risks (Liability)	High; Unlimited personal liability	Medium to high	Low; Generally, stock-holders are not liable, but the corporation is	Low; Generally, stock-holders are not liable, but the corporation is	Medium; Members have limited liability	Generally the same as a corporation
Business Taxes	Federal, state, county, and city	Federal, state, county, and city	Federal, state, county, and city	Federal, state, county, and city	Federal, state, county, and city	Federal, state, and property tax-exempt
Documentation Requirements	DBA unless it is under your own name; EIN if employees; Business license and seller's permit if products; County/city permits	DBA, EIN, business license, seller's permit, county/city permits, and written agreement advised	DBA, EIN, business license, seller's permit, county/city permits, Articles of Incorporation Bylaws	Same as corporation, but elect subchapter S corporation	DBA, EIN, business license, seller's permit, county/city permits, Articles of Organization	Tax exemption, Articles of Organization, Federal/state EIN (unless foundation or fund)
Limitations	One owner; All legal and operational responsibilities; Dissolves upon death; Higher risks	Share profits; Individually and jointly liable; Can be complicated; State restrictions may exist	Complicated paperwork; Extensive regulations, tax, and time; State to state variances; State restrictions may exist	Paperwork similar to corporation; State restrictions may exist	Limited personal liability; State restrictions may exist	Must abide by IRS requirements and operating provisions; Reinvest monies/donations into mission of charity

Additionally, you may want to meet with a local accountant, lawyer, or small business consultant to learn about local county or city business laws, regulations, and requirements. Most state, county, and city agencies have Web sites that are very informative and contain telephone numbers for direct contact and information. Gather all of the documents together and begin to formulate your legal structure choices by first meeting federal and state health care laws and professional practice regulations, and second, meeting federal and state business laws and regulations. You can always start out as one type of legal structure and then file documents at a later date to become another type as you expand or have more resources. Obtaining professional liability insurance and other necessary business insurance coverage is very important to minimizing business and professional risks.

Tips and Tools

You may be required to join a provider network either by a payer or by managed care organizations for the main purpose of keeping costs down. Provider networks are organizations of health care providers who render care to contracted individuals under certain terms. They perform contract negotiations on behalf of the member provider to the insurance payers, and may also perform value-added services such as marketing, continued education courses, and advocacy. Some require the provider to send their claims through them and charge a percentage of the reimbursement (volume of patients) to cover administrative fees. There may also be a yearly membership fee.

There are presently over 30 provider networks for private practitioners across the United States, each of them servicing different types of settings and membership requirements. Usually there is an application and credentialing process.

The advantages of belonging to a network include increased utilization by existing contracts or new contracts, increased assurance of timely payment, increased practice tools, increased practice education, and increased administrative support. The disadvantages are as follows: costs, no guarantee of increased patients, a possibility of crowding out of higher paying patients, a true increase in affiliation revenue, and a possibility of losing independence if in a binding agreement.

Make sure to read all of the fine print and ask lots of questions. Spend some time asking other practitioners about their experience with belonging to a provider network and comparing the services and costs of each of them. In summary, provider networks are the "middle man" who establishes the contractual relationships between you and the insurance companies. This does not apply if you are a nonprofit or cash-based business.

STEP 3: CREATE YOUR ORGANIZATIONAL STRUCTURE

Now that you have a general idea of what legal structure best corresponds with your rehab business concept, it's important to visualize and identify whom and how they will fit into your business structure. The *organizational structure* is the organization's outline of ownership, management, operations, and lines of authority. By developing your organizational structure, you create clear lines of organizational responsibility and communication, and accomplish your mission statement objectives.

✤ *Define the Three Basic Organizational Structure Components*

Creating your organizational structure is dependent on recognizing 3 basic components to business organizations[1]:
1. *Management*: Persons who commonly own or control the business operations and/or supervise employees.
2. *Operating core*: Persons (employees) who perform the actual hands-on work, such as staff therapists providing therapy services.
3. *Support services*: Persons (employees) who perform supportive work services or tasks for the operating core and/or management, such as the office assistant.

These three organizational components depend on defining operating roles and organizational types as they relate to both tax and legal structure, and health care laws and regulations. Management tasks are typically delegated to the rehab practitioner who has the authority to make clinical decisions and supervise or provide clinical leadership. Generally speaking, those management positions are filled by licensed or certified therapists and not therapy assistants in order to comply with the standards of practice. Operating core services and support services are performed along supervisory and standards of practice guidelines. These services are typically performed by staff therapists, therapy assistants, and aides, respectively, and are divided into client-related tasks and non–client-related tasks.

Depending on your legal structure choice, you may have to perform several organizational components at once: owner, chief operating officer or member, manager and supervisor, department head or director, staff therapist, and bookkeeper. For example, if you are a for-profit sole proprietorship rehab professional with no employees, then you will be performing as an owner and manager, operating core, and treating therapist, and you will be fulfilling all support services such as acting as your own secretary or medical biller and any other roles necessary to operate your rehab business. In another example, if your business concept is to be a nonprofit corporation, then you could be fulfilling the operating roles of the stockholder/owner, president, fundraiser, therapist, volunteer worker, and other positions required or needed to meet tax and legal structure guidelines and business operations.

To assist you in aligning the three organizational structure components to lines of authority and supervisory regulations or guidelines, fill in the Organizational Structure Plan Worksheet below. Personnel and their job responsibilities are dynamic business processes. These answers may change by the time you complete your business plan and implement your rehab business structure. However, planning your organizational structure now provides a systematic approach to facilitating your mission and vision statements, reconfirming your tax and legal structure, and promoting successful rehab business management.

If you already have a rehab business, use this worksheet to reaffirm your present organizational structure.

Organizational Structure Plan Worksheet

What is your tax structure?   ❏ For-profit   ❏ Nonprofit

What is your legal structure?   ❏ Sole proprietorship   ❏ Partnership   ❏ Corporation   ❏ LLC

What operating roles need to be filled?

❏ Owner/owners   ❏ Stockholders

❏ Partners   ❏ Board of directors

❏ Members   ❏ Officers (president, vice president, etc)

What operating roles can you (OT, PT, OTA, PTA) perform according to federal and state professional health care practice laws or guidelines?

❏ Owner/owners   ❏ Stockholders

❏ Partners   ❏ Board of directors

❏ Members   ❏ Officers (president, vice president, etc)

Who will perform the organizational components necessary for your rehab business concept?

1.   Management: _____

2.   Operating core services: _____

3.   Support services: _____

✛ Draw Your Organizational Chart

An *organizational chart* is the hierarchal and pyramidal graphic representation of the three organizational components. Commonly, it is referred to as a "flow chart." There are several different models (types) of organizational charts, but for our purpose, we are going to assist you in creating the flow chart that represents your business structure. Creating a flow chart is important to depicting the chain of command and, subsequently, assisting in role delineation and responsibilities.

The flow chart starts from the top of the page and continues to the bottom. Those persons with the most control and authority (management or supervisory roles) are put at the top, usually inside rectangular-shaped boxes. This is the first organizational structure component—management. The other positions from your Organizational Structure Plan Worksheet are created below the owner or manager according to next highest authority and supervisory responsibility. This would represent the operating core services. Support services could report directly to the owner, such as an accountant, or to someone in operating core services, such as an aide. Adjacent boxes depict consultants or other entities that advise or interact directly with the owner or top decision maker. Examples have been given.

Sole Proprietorship

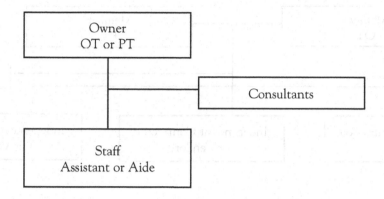

Partnership

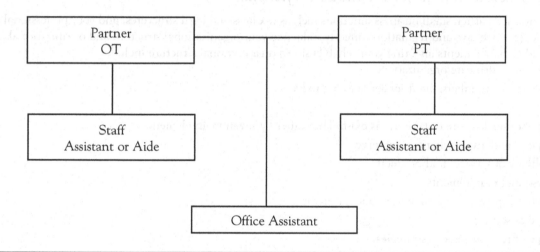

Corporation

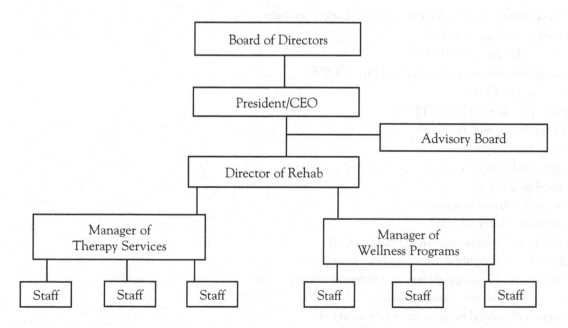

Limited Liability Company

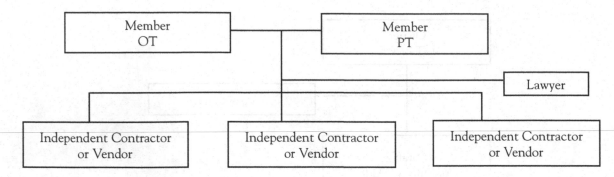

Special Considerations for the Rehab Professional

As mentioned earlier, small business functions such as tax laws and legal structures, and your professional standards of practice, practice law, and regulations directly influence your organizational structure and organizational chart.

Two additional elements affecting your rehab business organizational structure include:

1. Type of health care organization
2. Payment or reimbursement for services or products

Many types of health care organizations exist. They differ by seven main elements:

1. Type of patients or clients they serve
2. Delivery of services and products
3. Personnel requirements
4. Ownership type: government, public, or private
5. Type of setting
6. Type of reimbursement strategies
7. Accreditation and certification requirements

Some of the different types of health care organizations include:

*   Skilled nursing facility (SNF)
*   Home health agency (HHA)
*   Comprehensive outpatient rehab facility (CORF)
*   Rehab agency (RA)
*   Private practice (PTPP, OTPP)
*   Assisted-living facility (ALF)
*   Consulting company
*   Educational company
*   Home-based company
*   Community-based company
*   Contractor/subcontractor
*   Public health/welfare agencies (PHA/welfare)
*   School-based/nonpublic agency (school-based)
*   Voluntary health/nonprofit agency (nonprofit/charity)
*   Clinic/group practice (group practice)
*   Community mental health center (day centers)

- Durable Medical Equipment (DME)
- Federally qualified health center (FQHC)
- Hospice
- Outpatient services (Outpt OT/PT)

If you choose to become one of these organizations, keep in mind that they require a specific tax status and legal structure, and may require a specific organizational structure. As an example, CORFs mandate that certain rehabilitation professionals and services are hired and provided at one location. Certain health care organizations or state's standards of practice may also require additional accreditation, certifications, or post-educational training, and specific operational guidelines such as particular documentation and personnel supervisory guidelines.

There are advantages and disadvantages in each health care organizational type. The Department of Health Services (DHS) in each state generally provides information, applications, and external oversight to most organizational types listed. Contact them directly for documentation and forms. Both the state and national occupational and physical therapy associations and their member services are excellent informational resources to assist in determining what organizational type(s) your rehab business concept may fit into. You should also consult with other rehab professionals or health care experts to better understand the various parameters of the types of organizations.

How you will get paid for your services also affects your organizational structure. Government-funded health programs such as Medicare or Medicaid have regulatory policies and external oversight reviews and accreditation. If you decide to accept federal (www.cms.hhs.gov) or state health care funds (contact your state's DHS) for payment of services or products, you will need to apply and comply with the federal or state regulations or requirements. Furthermore, the supervisory roles of rehab professionals must also comply with federal guidelines. For example, your state's licensure language may state that the licensed OT and PT may supervise one OTA and PTA, respectively, and two therapy aides, respectively. However, if you are a sole proprietorship with employees that applies to Medicare as a private practice and, therefore, receives reimbursement from the federal government for services rendered to a Medicare recipient, you will need to follow Medicare's supervisory requirements. This may prohibit the use of an aide for client-related tasks. In most cases, the federal government has stricter organizational requirements than the state government or other agencies such as third-party payers. Therefore, your organizational structure and chart become flexible communication and working tools to your business and employees to satisfy necessary compliance rules.

Tips and Tools

For more information and software in creating your organizational chart, visit www.smartdraw.com. SmartDraw also provides software for business documents, floor plans, medical and anatomy posters, and other business templates.

For more information about various health care organizational types, visit the following Web sites:

- Center for Medicare and Medicaid Services: www.cms.hhs.gov
- American Occupational Therapy Association: www.aota.org
- American Physical Therapy Association: www.apta.org
- National Adult Day Services Association: www.nadsa.org
- Hospice Foundation of America: www.hospicefoundation.org
- Assisted Living Federation of America: www.alfa.org
- The Pennsylvania Rehabilitation Council: www.parac.org
- National Association of Rehabilitation Providers and Agencies: www.naranet.org
- Information for and about nonprofit organizations: www.npguides.org

STEP 4: SELECT YOUR BUSINESS NAME

Choosing a business name sounds like the easiest and most creative business step you have to perform, but, of course, there are legal requirements and necessary research tasks involved. You may have already noticed that tax and legal forms will ask for your business structure "name." However, the forms vary between federal, state, and local agencies, and so does the legal meaning of "business name." With the advancement of global technologies, the Internet, and the number of small businesses, finding a business name not already being utilized may be more difficult than you think.

Keep in mind that the legal structure you select affects which business name(s) you can choose from. Obtain expert advice from an attorney or small business consultant before making your final selection. Make sure you include necessary legal abbreviations such as LLC or Inc, if applicable.

✛ Definitions of Business Name Terms

Business name terms become increasingly more complicated and more important to understand as the legal structure and your business operations become more complicated. Business name clarification is needed to provide the numerous governing agencies, business organizations, and the public a clearer representation of your business.

Your business name(s) will also be used to market your services or products to the public and other health care providers, so take your time in selecting a name that will describe, entice, and be flexible enough for future business growth. Usually in health care, rehab professionals choose a name that signifies the type of services they are providing (eg, "Camarillo Aquatic and Rehabilitation Services").

Definitions of the main business name terms include:

- *Fictitious Business Name of (DBA, Doing Business As):* The name you will be conducting business under. For example, therapist A conducts business under her company called "Ultimate Rehab," which is the DBA. You register your fictitious business name with the County Clerk Registrar Recorder office in the county where your business is located. If you decide to use your own name, you may not have to register it. Check with the registrar office.

- *Legal corporate and company name:* The name you choose to incorporate and register with the Secretary of State. This name officially represents who owns the business and the legal structure. In my previous example, Ultimate Rehab is the name that business is conducted under. Ultimate Rehab, LLC is the official LLC name that represents the legal structure type, just as LLP or Inc represents a limited liability partnership or corporation, respectively.

- *Domain name:* The "Web address" that someone types in on the World Wide Web or Internet to find information, services, and products about your company. Our Web site address or domain name is www.ultimaterehab.com. You will need to register your domain name with an online service company such as www.namebuy.com or www.networksolutions.com.

- *Trademark:* The name given to any word, phrase, design, symbol, or logo used to market services or products (eg, a famous trademark is the golden arches of McDonald's or a famous phrase is Nike's, "Just do it"). You need to register your trademark with the U.S. Patent and Trademark Office (www.uspto.gov). If your business develops a logo, product, or phrase and you don't want anyone else to use it, take the time to register it.

✛ Research Your Business Name

Before filing or registering any business name, you will need to research whether it is available. There are several areas in which you should conduct your search. If you are using your own name and you plan to form a partnership or LLC, you still need to search for availability. Remember, there are many common names. Searching for your business name online is fastest and easiest. Ideally, it's easier to utilize the same business name in all aspects of registration that will meet local, state, and federal guidelines, so search for a business name that is available in all databases.

First, write down all of the business names you are thinking about. Next, depending on your legal structure, you will need to search all or just some of the places mentioned below. Don't register any business name until you have exhausted the search. Indicate those databases you searched next to the business names you selected (eg, Ultimate Rehab was available in all five databases below).

Business Name: _____ (a)____ (b) ___ (c) ____(d) ____(e) ____
Business Name: _____ (a)____ (b) ___ (c) ____(d) ____(e) ____
Business Name: _____ (a)____ (b) ___ (c) ____(d) ____(e) ____

City Databases (a)

Local Chamber of Commerce, Telephone Directories

Your local chamber of commerce and the phone directories are the first and easiest places to look up your business name selections. Type in "chamber of commerce, (the name of your city), (name of your state)" in a Web site search engine. For example, type "chamber of commerce, Los Angeles, California" to get quick, direct access to information. Or, go to the phone directory and find the phone number to the chamber of commerce office (it is usually found in the front section of the phone book). Don't forget to actually look up your business name ideas in the white pages and yellow pages. Did you find your business name listed? If yes, then you will need to choose another name.

County Government Databases (b)

Registrar-Recorder/County Clerk's Office

This office is where you register your fictitious business name. It can usually be found online or in the telephone book. To locate the County Clerk office online, go to a search engine and type in the name of your county and the name of your state. For example, for the County Clerk office in Los Angeles, California, type in, "Los Angeles County, California." Once in the county Web site, look for the Office of County Clerk, "doing business with us," "naming your business," or "fictitious business name." There will be a place where you can search their database for name availability. Type in one of the business names you selected above and see if the search locates a matching business name. If the search results in "no matching records," that business name is available. You may have to call the Office of County Clerk if a database is not available online. Is your business name available?

State Government Databases (c)

Secretary of State Office

This office is where you register your partnership, corporation, or LLC. To find this governmental office on the Internet, go to www.state.(abbreviation of your state).us. For example, to find the Secretary of State for California, you would type in www.state.ca.us. Click through until you find Secretary of State office information. Some states will offer links through pages to "starting a business," which will allow you to research for business name availability from their database of registered corporations, partnerships, or LLCs. You can also go to the yellow pages of your local telephone book, or look under the "state government" white pages for the telephone number to the Secretary of State Office. Call and ask for assistance in searching your selected business name availability in their business registration database. Is your business name available?

Federal Trademark Databases (d)

Federal Trademark Office

Even though you may not want to register a trademark name, you should search here also. This eliminates any future possibilities of infringement in case you change your mind. Trademark register is found under the U.S. Patent and Trademark Office. The database contains all federally registered and pending trademark names. Go to www.uspto.gov and choose "trademarks." You can search the trademark database for your business name idea. If no one has registered your name or any part of the name, the search will tell you "no matches found." However, if the name or parts of the business name are registered, you will receive a page of all related business names. You can click on one of the names to see who the business/company is, where they are located, what date the trademark was filed or granted, and a brief description of the company who owns that business name. For example, type in "wellness international." You will see several companies who have registered a name with "wellness international" in the title. Obviously, that name is not available, so begin the process of choosing another.

The World Wide Web Databases (e)

The Internet contains many search engines, such as Google or Yahoo. You can type your business name into the search location and quickly see whether any Web sites are listed. You can also go to www.networksolutions.com and type in your selected business name(s). You will notice that there are now several different types of extensions, such as .net or .info, which gives you opportunities to search and register the business name in several ways. There are basically no rules governing how your business name appears on the Internet, unlike when you register your name with the local, state, and federal governmental offices. You don't need to include "Inc" or "LLC" in your domain name. However, you want people to easily find and remember your domain name for easy access to your company's information on services and products, so choose a name that is the same as your business name or a close look-alike. For example, type in "Ultimate Rehab" at the web site mentioned above. You will see that "Ultimaterehab" is unavailable because it is already registered. Is your business name available?

Special Considerations for the Rehab Professional

The choice of your business name is very important. Your rehab business concept will need a business name that appeals not only to yourself, but also to your potential clients, your referral sources, and the community in which you will be located. It should also represent your services or products. Several ideas include:

- Your own name and professional title (eg, Sunday's Physical Therapy)
- Words that identify your services or specialty area (eg, Ergonomic Specialists, Inc)
- Words that represent your products (eg, Hands Only Rehab Products)
- Words that identify your organizational type (eg, Reminisce Day Care Center)
- Words that represent a location (eg, Westside Wellness Coach, LLC)
- Words that create an acronym (eg, JOG, Inc—Jacksonville's Orthopedic Group)
- Words that express an overall concept (eg, Creative Play Children's Center)
- Words that represent nonprofit funding (eg, Wilson Foundation for Homeless Adolescents)

To illustrate the different ways your rehab business name can be defined, take the example given above—"Westside Wellness Coach, LLC." The "LLC" indicates that it is an LLC that performs wellness consulting services. You would register this company or legal (structure) business name with the Secretary of State. However, your fictitious business name would be "Westside Wellness Coach," if that is the name you are going to advertise to the public and appear on your business cards, letterhead, and so on. Your domain name, if available, could be www.westsidewellnesscoach.com or www.wswnc.com.

Tips and Tools

There are many online resources to assist you in everything from business name creation to business name registration. Here are a few:

- Online trademark services and business name information at www.tmexpress.com and www.trademarksetc.com
- Online service company for creating domain names at www.nameboy.com
- NameRazor is a computer software program for creating business names at www.creative-name-generator.com
- Legal filing of business names and companies at www.legalfilings.com and www.incorporate.com

CHAPTER 2 SUMMARY

Determining your business structure involves several important steps.

Step 1: Determine Your Tax Status
- What is your business concept from Chapter 1?

_____

- Indicate your tax status.
  ❒ For-profit   ❒ Nonprofit

Step 2: Determine Your Legal Structure
- Indicate your legal structure.
  ❒ Sole proprietorship   ❒ Partnership   ❒ Corporation   ❒ LLC
- Does your legal structure meet state professional registration or _licensing or certification laws and regulations?_
  ❒ Yes   ❒ No
- Does your legal structure meet federal, state, and local small business laws?
  ❒ Yes   ❒ No

Step 3: Create Your Organizational Structure
- Write down your management team members.

_____

- Does your organizational chart reflect your management, operating core services, and support services?
  ❒ Yes   ❒ No
- Does your organizational chart correctly reflect supervisory regulations or guidelines?
  ❒ Yes   ❒ No
- Does your organizational chart correctly reflect your legal structure?
  ❒ Yes   ❒ No

Step 4: Select Your Business Name
- What is your business name?

_____

- Is it available on all five databases?
  ❒ Yes   ❒ No

Action Plan
  ❒ Select tax status
  ❒ Select legal structure
  ❒ Create flow chart
  ❒ Select business name(s)

REFERENCES

1. Nosse L, Friberg D, Kovacek P. *Managerial and Supervisory Principles for Physical Therapists*. Philadelphia, PA: Williams & Wilkens; 1999.
2. Physical Therapy Board of California. Physical therapist assistants in the realm of corporation ownership. Available at: http://www.ptbc.ca.gov/forms_pubs/pta_corp_ownership.pdf. Accessed December 30, 2008.

SUGGESTED READING

American Occupational Therapy Association. "AOTA Private Practice Pamphlet." Bethesda, MD: American Occupational Therapy Association.

Epstein C, Jaffe E. Consultation: a collaborative approach to change. In: McCormack G, Jaffe E, Goodman-Lavey M, eds. *The Occupational Therapy Manager*. 4th ed. Bethesda, MD: American Occupational Therapy Association, Inc; 2003:259-283.

Internal Revenue Service. Checklist for starting a business. Available at: http://www.irs.gov/businesses/small/article/0,,id=98810,00.html. Accessed August 21, 2007.

Internal Revenue Service. Tax information for charities & other non-profits. Available at: http://www.irs.gov/charities/index.html?navmenu=menu1. Accessed December 30, 2008.

Kintler D, Adams B. *Independent Consulting: Your Comprehensive Guide to Building Your Own Consulting Business*. Holbrook, MA: Adams Media, Inc; 1998.

Pakroo JD, Repa BK. *The Small Business Start-Up Kit*. 4th ed. Berkeley, CA: Nolo, Inc; 2006.

Piersol C, Ehrlick P. *Home Health Practice: A Guide for the Occupational Therapist*. Bisbee, AZ: Imaginart International, Inc; 2000.

Pinson L, Jinnett J. *Steps to Small Business Start-Up*. 4th ed. Chicago, IL: Dearborn; 2000.

Santucci D. *Choice of Entity: S, C, LLC's and Partnership*. Roseville, CA: Professional Education Services, LLP; 2002.

SCORE. Choosing the right name for my corporation or limited liability company. Available at: http://www.score.org/leg_choosing_name.html. Accessed August 21, 2007.

SCORE. Understanding buisiness structures. Available at: http://www.score.org/leg_6.html. Accessed January 21, 2008.

Small Business Administration. Starting your business. Available at: http://www.sba.gov/smallbusinessplanner/start/index.html. Accessed December 30, 2008.

RELATED RESOURCES

IRS
Tax help line
(800) 829-1040

IRS
Forms and publications and free small business tax kit
(800) 829-3676

IRS
Tax assistance for small businesses, trusts, and others
(800) 829-4933

ELECTRONIC RESOURCES

www.allbusiness.com: Small business information and forms.

www.aota.org: American Occupational Therapy Associations.

www.apta.org: American Physical Therapy Association.

www.bizfilings.com: Biz Filings; online site for forming LLCs and corporations.

www.cms.hhs.gov: Centers for Medical Services; provider/supplier enrollment, laws, and regulations

www.incorporate.com: Online services about incorporations.

www.insurancenoodle.com: Business insurance information.

www.irs.gov: Internal Revenue Service.

www.legalfilings.com: Incorporating online services in any state.

www.nolo.com: Legal information, services, and products.

www.sba.gov: Small Business Administration.

www.score.org: Service corps of retired executives.

www.smartdraw.com: Software for creating business charts, diagrams technical drawings and documents.

www.startupbiz.com: Online information, tools and services for start up businesses.

www.tmexpress.com: Expert legal research and information about trademarks.

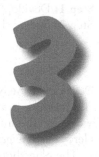

BUSINESS PLAN

Tammy Richmond, MS, OTRL

CHAPTER OBJECTIVES

✓ Develop your business plan.
✓ Secure the details.

Just as documentation of health care services or products is the fundamental and necessary task of all rehab professionals, the business plan is the fundamental and foundational document of a small business. It provides the rehab professional with a road map or blueprint to overall business operations.

Health care documentation consists of several components, all of which work together to facilitate and comply with standards of practice. Comparatively, the business plan contains several elements that work together to communicate and facilitate small business standards of operation.

A business plan can be defined as a "declaration of your goals and intentions, a written summary of what you aim to accomplish, and an overview of how you intend to organize your resources to attain those goals."[1]

There are two main objectives of a business plan[2]:
1. To describe the fundamentals of your business concept
2. To provide the financial calculations for lenders, investors, and successful business financial management

The first objective has three "internal" components[3]:
1. Define the vision, mission, goals, and objectives of the business concept.
2. Establish action plans and timetables.
3. Define consensus between decision makers on how to operate and grow the business.

The second objective has three "external" components[3]:
1. Persuade potential investors or financial partners.
2. Convince lenders to provide loans.
3. Convey to employees and the investors that the business has an organizational plan and direction.

There are two main steps to the business plan:

Step 1: Develop your business plan.

Step 2: Secure the details.

Step 1: Develop Your Business Plan

Developing the business plan will take lots of time and information gathering. You have already completed some of the initial work in the market research worksheet (see Chapter 1, pp. 13-14). You will build upon that worksheet to fully develop the information that is detailed in your business plan.

Here are some general rules to keep in mind:

- The plan should be about 20 to 30 pages long.
- The plan should be clear, concise, and easy to read.
- The plan should be as factual as possible.
- The plan should contain strengths, weaknesses, opportunities, and threats (SWOT).
- The plan should not contain rehab jargon language, unless it is defined.
- The plan should not contain highly confidential or proprietary information.[4]

✛ *Identify the Business Plan Components*

Business plan outlines vary depending on the industries for which they are developed, but, in general, a good quality business plan consists of three main basic components[4]:

1. Operations
2. Marketing
3. Financials

The operations component is a brief summary of the main elements of the day-to-day business activities. It can be compared to the treatment plan of health care (ie, a synopsis with short- and long-term goals). It includes your rehab business description, mission statement, location, management, financial status, long-term business goals, and a description of your products and services.

Marketing involves gathering information on the rehab industry and your specific area of practice, profiling the clients and potential clients for whom you want to provide services and products, assessing local competition, and developing promotional marketing strategies to communicate the benefits of your services and products. You will learn how to basically complete the marketing component here in this chapter, but you should wait to write the final marketing component until after completing the marketing plan in Chapter 4.

If you are developing your business plan in order to seek outside funding, the financials component is very important. Lending institutions need to feel comfortable with your ability to perform successful financial management before giving you any money. Generally, they will request certain financial documentation with projected or real income and expense costs. You should consider obtaining the skills and expertise of a small business accountant, financial advisor, or small business consultant.

Each of these components consists of several key elements. You will need to determine and define each of the elements in your business plan as best as you can. Some of the information will be exact, and some will represent your goals and intentions based on supportive research discovery. Your business plan will serve as a dynamic, flexible document that you will need to revisit often at the start, then at least annually once your business is up and running. Use the Business Plan Worksheet in Appendix A to write your own business plan. See the next page for an example of a business plan outline.

Business Plan Outline

Cover Page
Name of business
Name of owners
Addresses and phone numbers
Date of business plan prepared and by whom
Confidentiality statement

Executive Summary
Brief 2- to 3-page collections of paragraph summaries of the main business plan elements

Table of Contents

Operations
Business description
Mission statement
Management
Location
Products and services
Financial status
Long-term goals and *exit plan*

Marketing
Industry description and trends
Target market(s)
Competition
- Primary
- Secondary
- Advantages and strategic opportunities
- Risks and obstacles
Marketing strategies

Financials
Start-up costs
Operating costs
Income statement
Cash flow projections
Break-even analysis
Balance sheet
Sources and use of funds

Appendix of Support Documents
Résumés
Legal contracts
Legal agreements
Facility plans
SWOT analysis or other research analysis
Marketing materials
Supportive articles or other informational materials
List of business consultants, attorney, and accountant
Letters of reference

✦ Cover Page

Complete the necessary information for the cover page.

- Name of business: _____
- Name of owners: _____
- Addresses and phone numbers:_____
- Date: _____
- Prepared by:_____
- Confidentiality statement: _____

Example of a Cover Page

(Cover Page)

Business Plan

For

ABC Rehab, LLC

(Name of Owners)
(Addresses and phone numbers)
(Date)
(Prepared by)

This plan contains information that is proprietary and confidential to ABC Rehab, LLC. This obligation of confidentiality shall apply until such time that ABC Rehab, LLC makes the information contained in this business plan available to the public.

✦ Executive Summary

Although presented in the very beginning of any business plan, the executive summary is completed last. It serves as an overview of the business plan elements and answers such key business questions as:

- Who are you?_____
- What are your missions and goals? _____
- What are your services and products?_____
- Who are your clients (primary and secondary target markets)? _____
- What needs do your services (or products) satisfy? _____
- Who is your competition?_____

- What is your ultimate long-term goal?_____
- What is your exit strategy (expand, merger, buy-out, franchise, go public)? _____
- What is your financial status?_____
- Who is your management team (or owners)?_____

  The executive summary is sometimes the only document read by potential financial investors, lenders, or partners. Make sure it tells the reader what need will be filled, and where, how, and why your business concept will fill that need and be successful. Concentrate on your business concept's strengths and opportunities, your experience, and your unique services. Completing the remaining business plan elements will assist in writing the executive summary.

Example of an Executive Summary

Executive Summary

The Company

ABC Rehab, LLC, consultant specialists in rehab practice and management, was formed in 1998 by John Doe, PT, member, Chief Executive Officer, and Jane Doe, OT, member, Chief Operations Officer. The headquarter office is located in Paradise, United States. ABC Rehab's mission is to provide comprehensive practice and management consulting services and products in rehabilitation and wellness to occupational and physical therapists (OT and PT) working in the United States.

The Concept

Our goal is to create an online Web portal, www.abcrehab.com, for both OT and PT practitioners and health care consumers. We intend to establish both b-to-b and b-to-c content and commerce, member, and nonmember services. Our business model will enable us to:

- Provide real time integration of health care services between the practitioner and the consumers.
- Increase the convenience, speed, and quality of daily service operations.
- Provide integrated front and back office suite solutions.
- Allow easy access to health services and information.
- Integrate services with products.
- Integrate information from practitioner to practitioner.
- Integrate/comply with new governmental regulations and standards of practice.
- Detect emerging markets.
- Provide health care education, services, and products to the underserved consumer.
- Empower the consumer to monitor and track his or her health care.
- Empower the provider to redefine traditional delivery of health services.

  We believe that it is viable to create a network solution containing all of the necessary components to completely operate a rehab business and simultaneously create an online consumer population, providing them with educational home management. www.abcrehab.com will contain up-to-the-minute rehabilitation and health news, research, information, programs, services, supplies, data transferring, office solutions, support, and much more. Our dual business model will be able to dynamically change as health care changes, while integrating services and products as they are envisioned to be needed by the health care practitioner and consumer.

Products and Services

www.abcrehab.com will provide a comprehensive menu of rehab services and products that includes a Web-enabled back office practice management suite to chat rooms. Please see "Company Description: Products and Services" for a complete list. In addition, we will incorporate e-based and land-based site and information support, as well as sales consultants. Our Web site portal technology will allow easy, multiple access points from anywhere in the country.

(continued)

The Market

8 million people go online every day for health information (2006). An expected $2.8 trillion will be spent on health care overall by 2011. The existing online companies have positioned themselves mainly with physicians, pharmaceutical, and medical supply industries.

Rehabilitation and allied health professionals, along with other ancillary wellness providers, have been completely neglected in the e-healthcare industry. Moreover, no one has found a solution to educating and providing services to the growing number of underserved and uninsured consumers, and the OT and PT that service them.

Target Market

Our primary provider member and nonmember markets are OT, PT, and alternative therapy practitioners, who presently or in the future will provide reimbursable rehabilitative and wellness services and products.

Our primary consumer market includes the 8 million adults online every day searching for health info, the over 21 million who will visit their PT this year, 62% of Americans who are using some form of CAM, and the remaining visits to the other allied health professions that are not statistically accounted for. Our secondary consumer market is the underserved and underinsured who are unable to receive services either by lack of available OT and PT or by lack of financial resources.

The Competition

Currently, there is no dominant company serving the rehabilitation and wellness industry on the Internet. The few existing companies have focused on one or two practice management components. None of these sites are targeted for the health care consumer or are inclusive of private practice allied health professions and alternative therapies. In addition, none of the existing Internet companies seem to be envisioning the necessary business model to redefine the traditional delivery of services that will be required to meet underserved consumers, health care provider's basic practice management needs, and the continuous increasing number of online consumers looking for health and wellness education and resources.

Management

John Doe PT, CEO, and Jane Doe OT, COO, the founders of ABC Rehab, LLC, bring years of clinical and managerial expertise and experience in various aspects of rehabilitation and wellness. Both have worked within all types of health care settings and private practice. We will need to fulfill positions of CFO, (2) office staff, and (5) regional practice management consultants as funding allows.

The Future

Long-term development calls for expansion into four main components:

1. Provider–member
2. Provider–nonmember
3. Consumer–member
4. Consumer–nonmember

The dynamic business model allows for financial growth in all four areas together or separately. Our exit strategy is to merge with a larger medical online service model in 10 years.

Financials and Funds Sought

ABC Rehab, LLC anticipates that phase one Web site build-out will include health care provider and consumer nonmember services to cost $350,000 and take approximately 6 months. That includes the customizing of a partnering ASP, of which we will need to eventually support MEMBER platform components through our present technical team.

Phase two would consist of ASP building or the strategic partnership of member platforms to allow secure back office practice management and small business functions for the health care provider, and secure documentation retrieval and delivery for member consumers. This would take approximately 6 additional months and an estimated $250,000.

Cash flow projection revenue models for a 3-year projection include 30% advertisement, 30% subscriber fee, 25% e-commerce, and 15% data mining. We foresee the need to identify strategic partners and affiliations to offset the media model costs, back office solutions suite, marketing, and technical needs.

✤ *Table of Contents*

The table of contents allows easy access to all of the detailed information contained in the business plan.

Table of Contents

✤ *Operations*

This section contains descriptive information about your business concept. It includes several items that you have already completed in Chapters 1 and 2: your mission statement, vision statement, legal structure, and organizational structure. Typically, you write the business description in a narrative form, conveying the organizational elements in a logical sequence.

Complete the operations preparation statements below to assist you in writing the business description.

Operations Preparation

- Legal business name: _____
- Legal structure type: _____
- Organizational type (if applicable): _____
- Domain name: _____
- Any other names that will be used: _____
- Mission statement: _____
  _____
- Business goals: _____
  _____
- Owners: _____
- Management members: _____
- Other key personnel: _____
- Location: _____

- Description of services or products: _____
  _____
  _____

- If you are an existing business, your company history: _____
  _____
  _____

- Financial status:_____
  _____

Example of a Business Description

CHAPTER 3

Business Description

The Business

ABC Rehab, LLC, the parent consultant company, specializes in rehabilitation practice and management solutions, is based in Paradise, United States, and has been serving health care providers for over 5 years. www.abcrehab.com is our new Internet portal.

We assist organizations in creating new and successful ways to:
- Improve the quality of patient care
- Streamline systems and operations
- Comply with health care laws and standards
- Manage financial risk
- Start new practices, programs, and services
- Recognize, anticipate, and act on trends

The Business Mission

Our goals are two-fold. First, to provide OT and PT consolidated and integrated rehabilitation, wellness health care practice management, and information through a Web portal, www.abcrehab.com. This will allow us to build long-term relationships with our health care providers through quality services, products, information, and support, and to become known as the premiere online, integrated network procurement site. We can assist health care rehab businesses in controlling costs while improving quality of care throughout the country. We support change, innovation, and small business goals in the revolution of health care today.

Secondly, to provide a comprehensive, quality, and value-driven Web portal site for rehabilitation and wellness consumers. Our goal is to educate and enhance the consumer's experience with OT and PT, to promote products, and to establish an innovative approach to allowing all people to receive health care services.

Products and Services

In the b-to-b health care provider member and nonmember component, www.abcrehab.com will provide both commerce and content. Products and services will include:
- Web-enabled comprehensive back office practice management suite
- E-medical records
- E-content
- E-communities
- E-online store
- E-auction of rehab/medical products and supplies
- E-CEU/university/distance learning
- E-network: libraries, directories, screening tools
- E-bulletin
- E-hosting
- Ask the expert (live chats, archive, FAQs)

(continued)

In the b-to-c member and nonmember component, www.abcrehab.com will provide both commerce and content. Products and services will include:

- UR rehab/wellness network card
- E-rehab medical record access/tracking
- Self-monitoring home programs
- E-communities
- Interactive rehab advisor and screening tools
- E-network: self learning centers, libraries
- E-commerce
- Chat rooms
- E-hosting

Development to Date

ABC Rehab, LLC was founded in June 1998 by John Doe, PT, and Jane Doe, OT. The land-based consulting company specializes in rehab practice and management solutions. www.abcrehab.com was developed in Spring 1999 as a brochure site of services. In April 2000, www.abcrehab.com was upgraded to a content delivery and minimal commerce Web site for occupational therapy and physical therapy rehab business owners.

Legal Status and Ownership

www.abcrehab.com will be incorporated in the state of Nevada. The parent company, ABC Rehab, LLC, will continue as the land-based consultant company to the Inc and will expand its operations to fit the needs of the Inc.

Financial Status

Funding of the LLC and Inc has come completely from the owners. The company has no debt and continues to operate daily. The company is now seeking $350,000 dollars to finance the first phase of the Inc. These funds will be used to build the ASP infrastructure; hire payroll, technical, and data teams and additional content and commerce staff; and expand marketing activities.

✛ Marketing

The elements of marketing support your business operations by:
- Clearly identifying your potential or existing clients (target markets) of your products and services
- Outlining your business competition
- Defining your business concept's strengths, weaknesses, opportunities, and threats (SWOT) as they relate to your clients and competition

Subsequently, you develop marketing strategies (eg, local advertisements and community promotions) that highlight the unique benefits of your business, meet the demands of the clients, and fulfill the clients' specific needs for your services and products.

As rehab professionals, we expect that all of our clients have something in common—a need for clinical evaluation, treatment services, and products. Furthermore, medical physicians typically refer clients to rehab. Therefore, the necessity of developing a marketing plan seems unimportant and unnecessary. However, don't let traditional health care delivery channels fill you with false security. Today's health care marketplace is competitive and far-reaching. Consumers have many choices for health care services and products, and they expect value for their time and money, even if you are billing third-party payers or the federal government. You are competing with everyone who provides similar business services and products.

The marketing component will define the basic key elements of the larger and more detailed marketing plan that you will develop in Chapter 4. Conducting the research on your industry, your potential clients, and your likely competitors now will allow a better understanding of why and how marketing will affect the success of your business plan.

There are four elements to marketing:
1. Industry description and trends
2. Target market(s)
3. Competition
4. Marketing plan and strategies

Industry Description and Trends

Industry description and trends is a detailed look at the overall industry in which you work, your specific professional trade, the factors that affect your trade, the professionals who provide services and products similar to yours, and the emerging opportunities.

To begin, you must recognize the bigger picture of the global market. There are four economic sectors[5]:
1. Service
2. Manufacturing
3. Retail
4. Distribution

Typically, rehab professionals work in the service sector of the health care industry. However, if your business idea is to manufacture and sell a new therapy product, you would identify yourself in the manufacturing and retail sectors. Identifying your economic sector allows you to understand past history, present conditions, and future projections of economic factors that can influence your business success. For example, if you plan on manufacturing and selling a piece of balance equipment that is made of wood and you find out that wood products don't have longevity and don't sell as easy to therapy clinics because they cost more to ship, then you may want to change the composition of your equipment to plastic or you will lose money and consumers.

The federal government conducts statistical research on economic sectors at:
- www.fedstats.gov
- www.govspot.com
- www.dol.gov
- www.ntis.gov
- www.census.gov
- www.who.int/en

Use your research findings to answer these questions:
- What economic sector are you? _____
- What do you know about your economic sector? _____
- What are the history, present conditions, and future possibilities?_____
  _____
  _____

Your "industry" is the specific area of professional trade within the economic sector. For example, your economic sector is health care service, and your industry is occupational or physical therapy. To be more exact, your industry could be occupational therapy with a specialty in pediatrics. It will be important that you research and understand not only your trade, but also any specialty interests that directly impact your rehab business concept. The national and state associations and correlating trade magazines usually conduct annual surveys on current therapy practice areas. Information on practice areas specific to your specialty interests or certifications is also available through the state and national practice committees. Look at historical and present survey data to fully appreciate your business industry's growth and potential opportunities or trends.
- What is your specific industry?_____
- What is the historic growth of your industry? _____
- What are the industry trends (providers, clients, products, and services)?_____
  _____

TABLE 3-1

Impact Analysis on Industry

Rate the impact factors as high, moderate, low, or none, and circle the adjacent corresponding letter.

External Impact Factors	*Rating*			
Federal and state governmental health care policies	H	M	L	N
Federal and state health care regulation	H	M	L	N
State licensure and regulatory requirements	H	M	L	N
Standards of practice	H	M	L	N
Emerging markets	H	M	L	N
Potential consumer's wants and needs	H	M	L	N
Economical environment	H	M	L	N
Referral sources	H	M	L	N
Reimbursement trends	H	M	L	N
Competition	H	M	L	N
Technology	H	M	L	N
Internal Impact Factors	*Rating*			
Legal	H	M	L	N
Business operations	H	M	L	N
Personnel	H	M	L	N
Administration	H	M	L	N
Marketing management	H	M	L	N
Financials	H	M	L	N
Human resources	H	M	L	N
Standards of care	H	M	L	N
Competencies	H	M	L	N
Customer service	H	M	L	N
Documentation	H	M	L	N
Billing	H	M	L	N

- What are the threats? _____
- What are the opportunities?_____

Several external and internal factors can affect your industry and trends. It is important to examine these influential economic conditions and how they may impact your business concept. For example, the federal government imposes capitated reimbursements on outpatient occupational and physical therapy services. If your business concept is to create a community wellness center that will provide senior services and you plan to bill Medicare, you will have to plan on limited financial gains. Therefore, you may have to investigate other reimbursement strategies to be financially successful.

Investigate how these factors will impact your business concept within your business industry using Table 3-1. Anticipating the high and moderate external and internal factors impacting your industry will assist you in understanding and describing your industry and its emerging trends. See the next page for an example of industry description and trends.

Industry Description and Trends

Online Health Care Consumers Increase

Eight million people a day go online for health care information. 72.5% of all households use the internet. Proliferation of the overall health sector, the growing online population, increasing Internet commerce adoption, and the emergence of online shopping for prescription pharmaceuticals, OTC drugs, vitamins, herbal supplements, and personal health care has resulted in $205.2 billion dollars spent for online/offline consumer health care goods. An expected $2.3 trillion will be spent on health care overall in 2008, with $65.1 billion spent on allied health services alone.

Developing Health Care Provider Online Services

With pressure from the government and consumers preferring to have their health care "provider" online (54% of consumers prefer online health to be given by their own doctor), the medical community is now adopting itself to the Internet. 91% of physicians indicated that they are now using the Internet for professional purposes. The intensive information requirements drive by managed care and the shift to delivering information at the point of service will further drive physicians and allied health and alternative professions to the Internet.

Open Competitive Health Care Market Trends

National trends in managed care benefit coverage analysis showed 46.9% of plans covering chiropractic care and 43.4% covering wellness, besides the traditional allied health professions. In addition, over 629 million visits were made to complementary and alternative medicine providers, while only 386 million visits were made to physicians. Still, 8 million people a day go online and search for health care information from a variety of sources. Although WebMD has proven to be the most popular online medical website, the online health care audience shows no certain allegiance to any one source for information surfing. Besides our national association websites, there are currently no Occupational or Physical therapy web portals that offer health care information about our services and products.

Threats to Industry Market

Because of economic downfall, along with rising health care costs and the failure of managed care to contain costs, the federal and state governments continue to decrease overall spending on Medicare, medical, Medicaid, and other insurance coverage. Rehab businesses will struggle to meet overhead costs with the lack of reimbursement options. Additionally, several state practice acts are prohibiting the use of lesser-paid therapy aids for clinical patient tasks, making it impossible to decrease salary spending.

Opportunities

The increased use of technology in the OT and PT marketplace will facilitate further learning and utilization of the PC and other mobile device technologies. Rehab businesses will discover that decreased documentation time and integrated office management will save money. www.abcrehab.com has a strong opportunity to develop a dominant position among rehab business owners.

Target Market

A target market is a selected group of consumers (market) that you have identified (target) that wants or needs and will benefit from your business products and services. Target markets have four common characteristics[5]:
1. Definable
2. Meaningful
3. Sizable
4. Reachable

You must be able to define your consumers, what they value enough to spend money on, how many will potentially buy your services and products, and how they will benefit from your services and products.

By now, you have already selected who you feel will benefit from your rehab business services and products. Answer these questions about your target market.
- Who will buy your services or products? _____
- Where do they live? _____
- How many do you think need and want your services or products? _____

- Why do they need your services or products? _____
- Why will they spend money on your services or products? _____
  _____
- Who will pay for the services or products?_____
- When will they choose to utilize your services or products?_____
  _____
- Describe your expected client. _____
  _____
- What needs are you fulfilling (the opportunity)?_____

Example of the Target Market Element of a Business Plan

Target Market

Market Description

ABC Rehab, LLC is headquartered in Paradise, United States, and services rehab business owners across the country through regional subcontractors and through the Web site, www.abcrehab.com. Rehab business owners are collectively found in all 50 states.

Market Size

Physical Therapists

- 173,000 employed PTs in 2006, according to the Bureau of Labor Statistics
- 60,000 employed PTAs in 2006, according to the Bureau of Labor Statistics
- An expected increase of 27% of Physical Therapists is expected by 2016.
- An expected increase of 32% of Physical Therapy Assistants is expected by 2016.

Occupational Therapists

- 99,000 employed OTRs in 2006, according to the Bureau of Labor Statistics
- 25,000 employed OTAs in 2006, according to the Bureau of Labor Statistics
- An expected increase of 23% of Occupational Therapists is expected by 2016.
- An expected increase of 25% of Occupational Therapy Assistants is expected by 2016.

Primary Target

Health Care Providers

Our primary target market is the rehab business private practice owner who is either an OT or PT. The estimated number is around 65,000 practitioners.

Ancillary professions that crossover into types of rehabilitation account for another roughly 356,000 professionals (eg, speech pathologists, dieticians/nutritionists, recreational therapists, athletic trainers, chiropractors, certified personal trainers). All of the professional types could potentially benefit from our online integrated health care portal.

Secondary Target

Health Care Consumers

Our primary target market in the consumer subscription membership is the uninsured, underinsured, and small business owners with less than 100 employees. There are roughly 46.6 million uninsured Americans.

Our secondary target market in the consumer non-membership includes the 8 million adults searching Web sites for health info daily, the over 20 million who will visit their PT this year, the 700 million plus visits to CAM providers, and the remaining visits to other allied health professions that are not statistically accounted for.

- In 2006, 1.83 million injuries and illnesses resulted in time away from work (Safety and Health Statistics) with the most common being sprains and strains, and most often involving the back.
- 46.6 million Americans are uninsured. The average American, however, uses $2700 worth of health care a year.

(continued)

Market Readiness

Increasing diversity of population, expanding health care choices, increased need to balance acute care and preventive tasks, and aging populations are some of the multiple factors most affecting health care for the future. The time and money spent delivering health care services are astronomical. Increasing regulations by the federal government to control costs yet deliver quality care are going to drive all health care professionals online or out of business.

The average physician charge to managed care per patient is $79. Actual HMO reimbursement is $43. Administrative costs to the physician per patient are $20, and overhead costs are $30. Net to physician is minus $7. Allied health professions face a similar financial crunch. 45% to as much as 55% of total costs per month of managed care revenue is spent on administrative and overhead expenses. With the emerging trend of managed care organizations covering alternative medicine and therapies, along with the multiple factors affecting health care services, providers and consumers alike are going to find themselves needing to grasp and integrate new models of health care delivery.

Opportunities

Clearly, there is a real need to provide rehab business owners with an online business model that can increase efficiency and decrease costs. Consumers, underserved and uninsured, will continue to seek out health care information online first before spending cash on services that can be avoided. www.abcrehab.com promotes the interrelationship between the rehab business owner and the potential consumer by providing education, screening tools, learning centers, and commerce.

Competition

As a rehab professional, have you ever wondered about your competition? Competition is anyone who is striving to effectively attract and obtain your target market for the benefit of financial or other gains. It is all individuals or businesses that promote and provide similar services and products.

There are two main categories of competition:

1. Primary
2. Secondary

Primary competitors are those individuals or businesses that directly affect your business operations based on customer perception factors and internal operational factors.[5] For example, a primary competitor is another rehab business two blocks away that also specializes in sports medicine injuries and rehabilitation.

Secondary competitors are those individuals or businesses that could indirectly affect your business operations, such as personal trainers providing core-strengthening programs at the local fitness center.

Use the Competition Survey Chart on the next page to identify your primary and secondary competition. Drive around a 5-mile radius of where you plan to locate your business and identify potential competitors. Check the telephone directories, local newspapers, and chamber of commerce for professionals or businesses that provide similar services and products. Collect brochures and newspaper ads and network with local residents and area businesses to gain an accurate perception of your competition. Fill in the Competition Survey Chart with your information.

The SWOT Analysis that you performed in Chapter 1 is a good tool to compare your rehab business with your primary and secondary competitors. Write the strengths, the weaknesses, the opportunities, and the threats as compared to the competition from your Competition Survey Chart. Summarize your findings into the competition element of your business plan (see p. 61 for an example).

Competition Survey Chart

Factors	Primary Competitor	Primary Competitor	Secondary Competitor	Secondary Competitor
Location				
Parking				
Services/Products				
Specialty Areas				
Hours of Operation				
Marketing Materials				
Perceived Image (qualified, good service, etc)				
Reimbursement (cash programs, insurance, etc)				
Referral Sources				
Type of Personnel				
Competence				
Innovative (new programs, etc)				

Comparative SWOT Analysis Chart

SWOT Analysis Chart	
Strengths	*Weaknesses*
(eg, are open 6 days a week)	(eg, competitor has better parking available)
Opportunities	*Threats*
(eg, can offer area businesses worksite ergonomic consultations and services that no one else is providing.)	(eg, another larger clinic 5 miles away)

Marketing Plan and Strategies

Marketing plan and strategies are the communication tools between your rehab business and your target market that you will identify more clearly in Chapter 4. Therefore, you should come back and revise your marketing strategies before drafting your final business plan. However, marketing strategy decisions can be made at this point based on your understanding of your target market and competition.

There are several objectives of marketing strategies:
- To create awareness of your services and products to your target market
- To persuade your target market to choose your business over your competitors
- To communicate the benefits of your services and products
- To build target market loyalty
- To subsequently make a profit

There are four types of promotional marketing strategies:
1. Advertising
2. Sales promotion
3. Public relations
4. Personal selling

Selecting which promotional strategies to employ depends on several factors:

- Target market
- Competition
- Strengths and opportunities
- Time
- Money
- State regulations[6]

The Competition

Competitors with www.abcrehab.com are existing online consulting companies with services and products in our health care industry (occupational and physical therapy). They provide the following types of services and products:

- Consulting services
- Listservs
- Products
- Seminars
- Regulatory information
- Management tools
- Articles
- Online home exercise programs
- Medical and health informational directories

Primary Competitors

Two primary competitors are well established in our industry. One competitor's online presence consists of only a brochure-type Web site with no interactive models of exchange between company and practitioner. The other competitor owns and operates a more in-depth online presence with interactive models of information, comprehensive array of Web link relationships to vital regulatory, and practice standards across several types of rehabilitation work settings.

Secondary Competitors

Several online rehab-based Web sites provide home management software with various packages of rehab-based exercises and handouts. They do not expand their services beyond this primary product line. Other competitors are Web-based medical informational directories in which the provider or consumer can search for articles, educational information, and other health-related materials. One is a publicly held company with good market share of physicians and online health care consumers. There is a subscription fee for certain areas of Web site services.

Advantages Over Competitors

No competitors are targeting only private practice rehab business owners or underserved and uninsured consumers. There is no competitor who has integrated rehabilitation, OT, and PT with potential consumers of their services and allowed interactive networking and educating.

Risks and Obstacles

Occupational and physical therapy rehab business owners are limited by time, money, fear of risks, and lack of incentives to integrate information technology into their business operations. Many of them don't belong to industry organizations or associations that allow easier access to networking business management trends and services.

Opportunity (in Comparison to Competitors)

www.abcrehab.com has a great opportunity to become the only source for online integrated health care management and practice services for the OT and PT practitioner and the consumers they serve.

Here is a list of typical promotional strategies. Select those that meet your marketing objectives based on your target market and competition supportive research. See below for an example of Marketing Plan and Strategies.

❏	Business cards	❏	Promotional giveaways
❏	Brochures	❏	Trade shows
❏	Letterhead and envelopes	❏	Free assessments
❏	Ad placements	❏	News releases
❏	Flyers	❏	Article writing
❏	Emails	❏	Meet with referral sources
❏	Direct mailings	❏	Prescription pads
❏	Networking	❏	Web site
❏	Free demonstrations	❏	TV/Radio
❏	Open house	❏	Other ideas_____

Marketing Plan and Strategies

ABC Rehab, LLC understands the needs of occupational therapy and physical therapy customers based on a history of consulting projects, contacts, and feedback. Our proposed service, www.abcrehab.com, is an outgrowth of identifying the best means to reach and meet the demands of private practice rehab business owners.

The health care consumer will continue to surf the Internet looking for answers to his or her health care needs as supported by market research. Computers and Internet usage continue to grow with the help of donations and purchases made to libraries, schools, coffee houses, and other community placements.

ABC Rehab, LLC defines its mission by using the campaign slogan, "One Stop Rehab Source, Health Solutions." It reflects our goal to be the premier comprehensive Web site for all practice and management needs of our practitioner consumer. It also allows the consumer to grasp the message that they will find all of the information they might need to make informed choices about their health and therapy needs.

Online Presence

Our technical team will situate www.abcrehab.com at the front of all search engines by strategic alliances, extensive Web channeling, and cutting-edge information technology. Marketing to search engines will allow our consumers to readily find us. Email marketing strategies, such as purchasing consumer lists, online advertisements, and direct email postcards, will allow us to readily tap into our existing target markets.

Marketing Strategies

ABC Rehab, LLC will primarily market by participation at state and national association conference trade shows, by advertising and writing articles in rehab industry magazines, and through direct mailings with selected client lists.

We aim to establish strategic alliances with some of our competitors by sales and commission relationships. Our product lines will be generated through vendor contracts and will be promoted strategically through shared distribution strategies. www.abcrehab.com is also open to outsourcing, co-branding, acquiring, or partnering with other existing companies that complement our vision. We realize that personalization, convenience, communicating, and monitoring our user base will allow us the end-to-end integration online.

Organization of Regional Consultants

It will be necessary to provide national customer service and promote regional customized back office practice and management solutions for our consumers. ABC Rehab, LLC will hire and train five regional ABC Rehab consultants to meet these needs and market our services and products.

Marketing Position

ABC Rehab, LLC forecasts a 3-year marketing plan that will propel www.abcrehab.com to the top 10 health care Web sites visited by consumers. The company projects a 5-year marketing plan to reach and obtain 30% of our niche practitioner market.

✦ Management

In Chapter 2, Step 3, you defined the organizational components, completed the Organizational Structure Plan Worksheet, and created your organizational chart. Now is the time to put all of this previous work into your business plan. If your business plan objective is mainly to define your business concept for internal operational purposes, then writing your management element will be a general, narrative description of each person's background and their job responsibilities, which should correspond to their position on the organizational chart. On the other hand, if the business plan objective is to gain funding, then a more detailed description of owners, managers, and other top-level positions is required. Include résumés of all of the management personnel in the appendix of the business plan. Lenders want to feel confident that the funding they may be providing is going into experienced and capable hands.

If you are a single owner-manager and have no business experience, the funding sources typically ask for several letters of reference and 3 to 5 years of personal income tax returns. They will conduct a credit check for outstanding debt and payment history.

If you are still choosing between legal entities such as a partnership or LLC versus a sole proprietorship or single-owner corporation, keep in mind the financial history of all owners (managers) is important to lending institutions. Be sure to address these issues before signing any legal contracts. One owner's bad credit history may be enough to prevent you from receiving the necessary finances to implement your business concept.

- List the key members of your management team:

  _____

  _____

  _____

- List any consultants, attorneys, or accountants:

  _____

  _____

  _____

- Collect résumés from all of the names listed above. You will utilize some of the information to write your management section and include copies of the résumés in your appendix.

If possible, include the organizational chart within the management section. Otherwise, include the chart in your business plan appendix. See the next page for an example of the management element of a business plan.

✦ Financials

Money is one of the most uncomfortable issues to deal with, regardless if you are making money or spending money. Certainly, if you are going to own and operate a rehab business, you will need to become familiar with all aspects of financial management. You will learn more in Chapter 6 (see Glossary for the definitions of financial terms).

Which financial documents you will need to complete is dependent on your business plan objectives. As a start-up rehab business, you may only be able to provide estimated start-up costs, operating costs, and cash flow projection because you have no business financial history as of yet. On the other hand, if you are starting a consulting business with a partner and will have an office location for business operations and meetings, you will need to pay rent, basic overhead expenses like office equipment, and maybe employ a part-time office assistant. Completing certain financial statements and forms will assist in determining if you need funding or how much each partner will need to contribute to meet start-up and operating costs. However, if you are opening up an incorporated clinic with several staff members and offering multiple services and products that require extensive equipment needs, you may have to apply for a sizable business loan. The lender will require more extensive financial documentation to base a lending decision on.

To decide on how much and what information you will need to complete the financials component, ask these four important questions[7]:

1. How much will it cost to implement my rehab business plan?
2. Will I need to borrow money?
3. If so, how much do I need, and when will I need it?
4. What different types of funding sources are available to me?

Realistically, you will be making educated decisions with real and predicted mathematical calculations based on financial research. You will easily know how much certain items cost, and for others, you will make the best "guestimation" available.

Management

Key Members

John Doe, PT, member and Chief Executive Officer

John has been a PT for more than 20 years. He has graduate degrees in management and business. Besides his partnership in ABC Rehab, LLC, John owns and operates a multidisciplinary outpatient clinic. He also works as an expert witness and has consulted on more than 100 legal cases involving rehabilitation. John holds a faculty position at the University of Higher Education, where he teaches health care administration to graduate and doctoral students. He is actively involved in the American Physical Therapy Association and the rehab community, holding local, state, and national offices. John owns 50% of the LLC.

Jane Doe, OT, member and Chief Operations Officer

Jane has been an OT for over 18 years. Jane works in various areas of health care, fitness, and wellness in her own private practice. Jane has authored several articles and developed a comprehensive fitness video series. Jane is actively involved in the American Occupational Therapy Association and several other professional organizations, and she lectures on various management issues. Jane owns 50% of the LLC.

K. Smart, Technical Team Manager and Coordinator

K is an information technology specialist. His company, Web Site Specialists, has developed several of the Fortune 500 companies' IT services. He brings with him a team of technicians with years of development and marketing experience.

Consultants

Mr. Attorney serves as the company's legal consultant. He specializes in health care on the Internet and has authored and lectured on e-healthcare industries around the country.

Mr. Accountant serves as the company's accountant. He specializes in small business tax and accounting, and will continue on an ongoing basis.

Advisory Committee

An Advisory Committee has been informally selected to provide guidance to www.abcrehab.com. The Advisory Committee will meet quarterly. Members of this committee are S. Medical Doctor, P. Nutritionist, L. Exercise Physiologist, and T. Speech Pathologist.

Management Structure

Jane Doe is involved in the day-to-day operations. She works directly with the technical team manager and will oversee outsourcing contracts with vendors and other affiliated organizations. John Doe is in direct communications with the advisory committee and attorney.

Management responsibilities are depicted in the flow chart below.

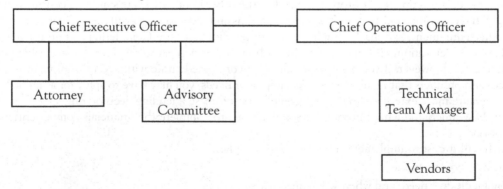

The goal of www.abcrehab.com is to build out into four online platform services areas; member and nonmember provider services and member and nonmember consumer services. The plan calls for two build-out phases. ABC Rehab, LLC acknowledges that a chief financial officer, a vice president of marketing, and additional advisory boards or boards of directors in each of the four areas in www.abcrehab.com will need to be added.

There are several different types of financial documents. Accounting software programs such as Quickbooks, Quicken, and Peachtree contain financial forms and other bookkeeping tools for easy use. These forms will be used as part of your financial management that you will learn about in Chapter 6.

Some examples of typical financial forms include:
- Start-up costs
- Operating costs
- Income statement (profit/loss)
- Cash flow projection
- Balance sheet
- Break-even analysis
- Sources and use of funds

In completing financial documents, keep these practical guidelines in mind[5]:
- Be conservative.
- Be honest.
- Don't be creative.
- Learn the terminology.
- Follow the practices in your industry.
- Choose the appropriate accounting method.
- Be consistent.
- Get an accountant's advice and assistance.

Start-Up Costs

The first step to building a sound financial plan is to devise a start-up budget. Determining the basic expenses for your rehab business start-up is a good place to begin. Do your homework and fill in the Start-Up Costs Report below as accurately as possible. Obtain assistance from online research. Call and interview associated agencies, companies, and rehab professionals in your area that correspond to the expense item.

Start-Up Costs Report

Items	Costs
❏ Personnel (costs prior to opening)	_____
❏ Legal fees	_____
❏ Lease/rent	_____
❏ Licenses/certification	_____
❏ Business licenses/permits	_____
❏ Equipment	_____
❏ Office furniture	_____
❏ Insurance	_____
❏ Office supplies	_____
❏ Advertising/promotions	_____
❏ Salaries/wages	_____
❏ Accounting fees	_____
❏ Consultant fees	_____
❏ Utilities	_____
❏ Professional membership fees	_____
❏ Business banking fees	_____
❏ Telephone/fax/Internet	_____

Operating Costs

Similar to start-up costs, operating costs are the expenses that will continue as monthly payments. For example, you paid for many hours of legal and accounting assistance to start your business, but you may not have any monthly legal or accounting expenses. Or, you decided to lease some equipment and purchase other equipment. The monthly lease will become a deductible operating cost and the purchased equipment will have a depreciation amount.

Operating costs or business expenses are divided into three categories:
1. Fixed expenses (costs)
2. Variable expenses (costs)
3. Purchase expenses (costs)

Fixed expenses (*costs*) are those business expenses that you pay regularly every month that do not directly relate to your services or products. Fixed costs are commonly called "overhead expenses." Items such as rent, telephone bills, utilities, insurance, professional fees, cleaning, and loan payments are examples of fixed costs. *Variable expenses* (*costs*) are those business expenses that can fluctuate according to demand and utilization (eg, office supplies, medical supplies, payroll expenses, and marketing expenses). Salaries and labor costs can be both fixed and variable depending on the employee status, such as a full-time salaried employee versus the independent contractor therapist who provides services. *Purchase expenses* (*costs*) are those costs that represent the expense items purchased for the rehab business. Fill in the Operating Costs Report below with real or realistic numbers.

Operating Costs Report

General Fixed Expenses	Costs
❏ Rent/lease	_____
❏ Utilities	_____
❏ Depreciation	_____
❏ Insurance	_____
❏ Loan repayments	_____
❏ Financial administration	_____
❏ Clinical salaries and wages	_____
❏ Office salaries and wages	_____
❏ Benefits	_____
❏ Office supplies	_____
❏ Professional fees/licenses	_____
❏ Laundry and cleaning	_____
❏ Telephone/fax/Internet	_____

General Variable Expenses	
❏ Marketing	_____
❏ Outsourcing fees	_____
❏ Salaries	_____
❏ Medical/clinical supplies	_____
❏ Maintenance and repair	_____
❏ Education	_____
❏ Travel	_____

General Purchase Expenses	
❏ Office equipment	_____
❏ Clinical equipment	_____
❏ Business automobile	_____
❏ Other_____	_____

Income Statement

Income Statement: Annual for 3 years	Year:	Year:	Year:
Income:			
Gross income from services or products			
Less bad debt and cost rate (outsourcing costs)			
Net income			
Costs of general fixed expenses			
Gross Profit:			
General Fixed Expenses:			
Salaries and wages			
Payroll taxes			
Benefits			
Equipment			
Maintenance and repairs			
Lease/rent			
Utilities			
Office supplies			
Telephone/telecommunicating			
Medical supplies			
Marketing			
Professional fees/licenses/permits			
Depreciation			
Total Expenses:			
Net income before taxes			
Provision for taxes on income			
Net Income After Taxes (Net Profit):			

Income Statement (Profit/Loss)

An income statement (also called "profit and loss statement") is generated to quickly look at your business concept profitability. Most often, lenders want to see a historical income statement (ie, one representing the company's yearly income and expenses for the past 3 to 5 years). If you are just starting, you won't have any business financial history to report. Instead, you will typically be asked to provide the last 3 years of personal income tax returns plus two or three letters of financial reference. A typical example of an Income Statement is provided above. The income statement categorizes your revenue and expenses, giving a general but complete overview.

Cash Flow Projection

A cash flow projection or pro forma cash flow statement is a financial document that forecasts what cash or income is being received and what cash is being paid out. If you are already in business for yourself, you will have numbers to use. If you are just starting, your projected numbers will be estimated based on real probabilities. In health care, unlike retail sales, income or cash flow can be delayed several weeks, especially if you are billing third-party payers or federal and state insurance funds. This is where some rehab business owners miscalculate. You can't pay for operational expenses if you don't have enough monthly cash (reimbursement) flowing in a timely manner. A general rule of thumb is to have enough funds to cover your start-up costs and operating costs for 6 months. This can provide you with a cash base just in case you miscalculate your monthly cash flow. See the next page for an example of a Cash Flow Projection for 1 Year chart.

Cash Flow Projection for 1 Year

Cash Flow: 1 Year	Jan	Feb	Mar	Apr	May	Jun	Jul	Aug	Sep	Oct	Nov	Dec
Opening Cash Balance												
Cash Receipts												
Accounts receivable												
Collections												
Loans/interest												
Total Cash In												
Cash Payments												
Start-up costs												
Rent												
Utilities												
Depreciation												
Insurance												
Loan repayments												
Lease payments												
Clinical salaries												
Office salaries												
Benefits												
Payroll wages												
Office supplies												
Medical supplies												
Postage												
Laundry/cleaning												
Telephone/fax/Internet												
Licenses/permits												
Professional fees												
Marketing												
Outsourcing fees												
Maintenance/repair												
Education/CEUs												
Travel												
Income taxes												
Misc												
Total Payment												
Opening Cash Balance												
Cash receipts												
Cash payment												
Ending Cash Balance												

Balance Sheet

The balance sheet is a financial document that provides a present snapshot of your rehab business' worth. It calculates your assets and subtracts your liabilities to show the net worth of your business at any given moment. Lenders, investors, or potential buyers will request this financial document to view the value of your rehab business. Expert assistance is recommended. See below for an example of a Balance Sheet.

Balance Sheet

Business Name: _____

Date: _____

Assets

Current Assets

Cash	$_____
Accounts receivable	$_____
Inventory	$_____
Prepaid expenses	$_____
Total Current Assets	$_____

Fixed Assets

Land	$_____
Building	$_____
Improvement	$_____
Equipment	$_____
Furniture	$_____
Automobiles	$_____
Less accu. depr.*	$_____
Total fixed assets	$_____
Other assets	$_____
Total Assets	$_____

Liabilities

Current Liabilities

Accounts payable	$_____
Short-term notes payable	$_____
Federal income tax	$_____
Self-employment tax	$_____
State income tax	$_____
Sales tax accrual	$_____
Property tax	$_____
Payroll accrual	$_____
Long-term liabilities	$_____
Total Liabilities	$_____

Net Worth (Equity)

Proprietorship	$_____
Partnership	
Name _____ , 51%	$_____
Name _____ , 49%	$_____
Corporation	
Capital stock	$_____
Retained earnings	$_____
Total Net Worth	$_____

*Less accumulated depreciation

Break-Even Analysis

The *break-even analysis* is the financial document that will determine how much income you will need to make to meet your business expenses. It incorporates your business operating costs, your break-even calculations, and your *operating income*. Subsequently, you will be able to generate a dollar amount or a "visits per day to break even" (see Appendix B) that represents your break-even point.[8] After the break-even point, you have profit. The break-even analysis can be complicated in a rehab business because it requires that you know usual and customary charges for your services, and the reimbursement percentages minus any outsourcing expenses.

Compiling the number figures for the break-even analysis also requires that you revisit the external and internal economic impact factors that were mentioned in industry description and emerging trends (see p. 56). These same impact factors will influence how you estimate income and expenses. For example, let's say that the state board of physical therapy has revised the licensure and regulatory policies to eliminate the use of aides for clinical, patient-related tasks. The law goes into effect in 6 months. Therefore, you will have to make revisions to the staffing salaries estimated on your break-even analysis to meet new legal requirements. It will cost more to staff in compliance with the law. Other factors, like Medicare and third-party reimbursement changes, will also affect your break-even analysis. It is impossible to be 100% certain of all of the numbers you compile, but attempt to be as accurate as possible. If you are going to present the business plan to lenders for funding, they will generally ask you how you obtained your figures. They will probably not be familiar with your rehab business, so you will need to convince them that you are confident in your financial calculations. Obtain professional assistance from small business or therapy consultants, accountants, and medical billing services, if necessary.

Sources and Use of Funds

If you have determined that your rehab business requires additional funding, or if you are a partnership, corporation, or LLC, a descriptive statement of how much money you need, what it will be used for, and who will supply the funds is important. The sources and use of funds statement is a great financial tool for clarifying financial resources, especially when there is more than one owner. Even if you are the sole contributor of your rehab business's financial needs, completing the sources and use of funds statement is a good exercise in financial management. If you hire an accountant, he or she will want to know how much money came out of your pocket or through personal loans to pay for your business expenses. An example of a Sources and Use of Funds Statement is given on the next page.

Special Considerations for the Rehab Professional

A common mistake with the business plan is to not spend enough time researching your target market (clients). There is a misguided assumption in health care that you already know the characteristics of the typical client, or that because you already have referral sources, you don't need to worry about whether you are meeting the needs of your clients or if they will come to you for services. This ill-advised assumption can lead to business failure. Make sure to take time to fully understand your target market and their real needs, not the ones you think they have.

Perform verbal or written surveys and talk with area colleagues, businesses, peers, and others to get a true sense of what services and products are viable. Don't forget to look at the external environmental impact factors, such as changing health care laws and insurance reimbursement strategies and trends.

Another common mistake is miscalculating your financial needs. Cash flow is vital to your rehab business survival. On paper, the numbers may make complete sense to you, but in reality, unforeseen costs can quickly erode away your cash reserve. Talk to other colleagues who are already working in their own rehab business. Ask them about operating expenses and other expenses that they may not have expected, such as local permits and business licenses. Spend the time with a small business accountant or consultant to determine the cash flow projection for 1 year as accurately as possible, and make sure you have enough money for the first 6 months

Sources and Use of Funds Statement

Business Name: ABC Rehab, LLC   Date: 1/01/04

Owners: J. Doe, PT, and J. Doe, OT

Total dollar amounts sought: $45,620.00 in equity funding. The business partners will contribute the entire amount. If the business decides to later expand, funding may be sought preferably by one investor or long-term loan.

Source of Funds

Equity Financing

Name: John Doe, member, CEO	51% equity	$23,266.20
Name: Jane Doe, member, COO	49% equity	$22,353.80

Use of Funds

Capital Expenditures

Leasehold improvements	$500.00
Purchase of equipment	$8000.00
Purchase of furniture	$2000.00
Other miscellaneous purchases	$500.00
Total Capital Expenditures	$11,000.00

Working Capital

Technical team staff	$2500.00
Web site package with yearly maintenance	$3000.00
Online banking fees for 1 year	$180.00
Domain name fees	$270.00
Marketing activities	$10,000.00
Part-time office staff	$15,000.00
Legal fees	$2500.00
Small business fees	$820.00
Accounting fees	$350.00
Total Working Capital	$34,620.00

STEP 2: SECURE THE DETAILS

The appendix section of the business plan should include all of the documents that you created, completed, or compiled to support the elements of the business plan. They include:

- Résumés
- Articles of incorporation and partnership agreements
- Legal contracts
- Facility blueprints
- Lease agreements
- SWOT analysis or other research analysis
- Marketing materials
- Supportive articles or other informational materials
- Financial documents
- Letters of reference

Example of an Appendix

Appendix

Supporting Documents

A.   Résumés of Management Team
B.   LLC Articles of Organization
C.   LLC Partnership Agreement
D.   Service Contract With Technical Team
E.   Office Lease Agreement
F.   Industry Web Site Statistics
G.   Target Market Analysis
H.   Competition SWOT Analysis
I.   Cash Flow Projections
J.   Income Statement
K.   Balance Sheet
L.   Break-Even Analysis
M.   Letters of Business Reference

Special Considerations for the Rehab Professional

There are some guidelines to presenting your business plan outside of your immediate business management team and personnel. Your business plan is your business. You have spent hours developing your business concept, and even if you think your services are typical rehab services, the manner in which you will operate and present your business services and products is not.

To ensure the confidentiality of your business plan, you should consider drafting a nondisclosure agreement. This agreement is generally not necessary for lending institutions, but for outside consultants or prospective employees of your company (ie, a program coordinator, medical biller, or independent contractor), a nondisclosure agreement prevents unnecessary information from circulating among other colleagues. Consult with an attorney if necessary. There are nondisclosure agreement templates available online or in small business documents books.

If you are going to present your business plan for financial assistance, make sure the business plan looks professional. Go to a copy center and have the business plan printed on quality paper and covered in professional binding. Make sure to include your logo (if you have one) on the cover sheet.

You should revisit your business plan at least annually or anytime you need to refocus your mission, vision, and business objectives.

Tips and Tools

If you are in a position of buying or selling a health care business or practice, the items that should be included in a practice appraisal include the following:

- Financial Statements: operating costs, break even analysis, etc.
- Revenue Share: income from insurance, income from cash, other income
- Number of Procedures per client per session
- Billing: EOBs; accounts receivable; % of Medicare, PPO, HMO, etc.
- Gross Per Month (last two years)
- Number of Clients per month (last two years)
- Number of New Clients per month (last two years)
- Number of Referring Physicians: types of MDs (internists vs. surgeons, etc)
- Staffing: how many, type of contract, length of contract, benefits
- Production Per Therapist per month (last two years)
- Current Payroll Journal (include position & hire date)
- List of Major Medical Equipment
- List of Office Equipment: leased or own?
- Appraisal of Equipment: both medical and office, the depreciation left, etc.
- Lease: how long, how much, when to be renewed, is this a lease assumption clause
- Estimate of Supplies on Hand
- Current affiliations

You should ask to sign a confidentiality agreement, and ask to be able to show these documents to a consultant, accountant, bank loan officer, or lawyer to assist you in determining the reality and the value of the business. Sellers typically don't sell their aging accounts, and you should not want to buy them. Ultimate Rehab, LLC can assist you in selling or buying.

CHAPTER 3 SUMMARY

Developing your business plan involves identifying the main components and their elements.

Step 1: Develop Your Business Plan
- What is your business plan objective? _____
- What are the three main components of a business plan?
    1. _____
    2. _____
    3. _____

Step 2: Secure the Details
- Did you conduct thorough research to support your business plan?   ❏ Yes   ❏ No
- Can you clearly describe your business concept?   ❏ Yes   ❏ No
- Can you easily describe your specific industry and emerging trends?   ❏ Yes   ❏ No
- Can you describe a typical consumer that will benefit from your services or products?   ❏ Yes   ❏ No
- Write down three advantages your rehab business has over your primary competition.
    1. _____
    2. _____
    3. _____
- Name three marketing strategies that you feel will reach your target market successfully.
    1. _____
    2. _____
    3. _____
- Which financial forms did you complete for your business plan?

    _____
    _____

- Did you reconfirm your money figures with an accountant?   ❏ Yes   ❏ No
- Did you include all of the necessary supportive documents in your appendix?   ❏ Yes   ❏ No
- Is your business plan less than 30 pages, easy to read, and factual?   ❏ Yes   ❏ No

Action Plan
 ❏ Write your business plan
 ❏ Secure the details with research, an accountant or lawyer, and documentation

REFERENCES

1. Sohnen-Moe CM. *Business Mastery: A Guide for Creating a Fulfilling, Thriving Business and Keeping it Successful*. 4th ed. Tucson, AZ: Sohnen-Moe Associates, Inc; 2007.

2. Nolo. Writing a business plan. Available at: http://www.nolo.com/lawcenter/ency/article.cfm/objectid/8AE4F799-0038-4471-B573659C196695D2. Accessed April 17, 2003.

3. Johannsen M. *Developing a Sound Business Plan*. Westlake Village, CA: Legacee Management Systems, Inc; 1995.

4. Page G. Chartered Management Institute: writing a business plan. In: *Business: The Ultimate Resource*. Cambridge, MA: Perseus Publishing; 2002:486-487.

5. Abrams R. *The Successful Business Plan: Secrets and Strategies*. Palo Alto, CA: Running 'R' Media; 2000:74.

6. Hertfelder S, Crispen C. *Private Practice: Strategies for Success*. Bethesda, MD: American Occupational Therapy Association; 1990.

7. Pinson L, Jinnett J. *Steps to Small Business Start-Up*. 4th ed. Chicago, IL: Dearborn; 2000.

8. Kovacek P. New practice analysis spreadsheet. Available at: http://www.ptmanager.com/starting_a_new_therapy_practice.htm. Accessed December 30, 2008.

SUGGESTED READING

American Occupational Therapy Association. Starting a Private Practice. Available at: http://www.otjoblink.org/links/link05.asp. Accessed December 30, 2008.

Ashley M. *Massage: A Career at Your Fingertips*. 3rd ed. Carmel, NY: Enterprise; 1999:57-74.

Berry T. The business you're in. Available at: http://articles.bplans.com/index.php/business-articles/writing-a-business-plan/the-business-youre-in/43. Accessed October 29, 2008.

Farrell S, Jaszcar A. How-to create a business plan. Available at: http://www.how-to.com/Operations/How_to_write_a_business_plan.htm. Accessed December 30, 2008.

Nosse L, Friberg D, Kovacek P. *Managerial and Supervisory Principles for Physical Therapists*. Philadelphia, PA: Williams & Wilkens; 1999.

Pakroo JD. *The Small Business Start-Up Kit (for California)*. 3rd ed. Berkeley, CA: Nolo, Inc; 2001.

Small Business Administration. Write a business plan. Available at: http://www.sba.gov/smallbusinessplanner/plan/writeabusinessplan/index.html. Accessed December 30, 2008.

ELECTRONIC RESOURCES

www.ahrq.gov: Agency for Healthcare Research and Quality; Medical Expenditure Panel Surveys.

www.allbusiness.com: Small business resources and documents.

www.bizjournals.com: Online business journal of tools, events, information.

www.bls.gov: Bureau of Labor Statistics; online statistics for many categories, professional, expenditures, etc.

www.cdc.gov: Center of Disease Control; health care library of topics, conditions, clinical trials, medical news, and research.

www.fedstats.com: Web portal for Federal Statistics; consumer expenditures, statistical information on demographics.

www.fundingsupport.com: Online site to assist you in securing funds.

www.govspot.com: Portal to websites of multi-agency health initiative and activities of the US Department of Health and Human Services and other federal departments and agencies.

www.leaseassist.com: Online site to assist you in negotiating commercial leasing.

www.nccam.nih.gov: National Center for Complimentary and Alternative Medicine and the National Institutes of Health.

www.npguides.com: Grant writing tools for receiving funding for non-profit organizations.

www.sba.gov: Small business administration.

www.score.org: Retired executives who counsel on small business topics.

www.startupbiz.com: Online information site for various start up business tools.

www.workingsolo.com: Small business support information for businesses with 20 employees or less.

MARKETING PLAN

Tammy Richmond, MS, OTRL

CHAPTER OBJECTIVES

✓ Analyze your market.
✓ Create a marketing plan.
✓ Implement your marketing plan.
✓ Assess and redirect your marketing strategies.

Marketing is a vital function to business survival, but it is often underutilized or misunderstood by rehab business owners. "Tell them what they get, not what you do."[1] This is where the marketing confusion begins. Marketing often gets misinterpreted as educating the doctors or the community on who you are or what you do and not what they get.

Marketing is "a social and managerial process by which individuals and groups obtain what they need and want through creating and exchanging products and value with others."[2] Marketing involves several activities "designed to sense, serve, and satisfy" the potential client, physician, or whomever you are targeting your message and efforts.[2]

The main objectives of marketing are as follows[3]:
- To identify and meet the target market's (customer's) needs and wants
- To create awareness of the product or service
- To increase accessibility to the consumer
- To persuade the consumer to purchase the product or service
- To meet the operational and financial business goals
- To build consumer loyalty based on value and satisfaction
- To achieve financial profits

In Chapter 3, you learned that marketing is one of the three components of a business plan. In fact, you identified your consumer target market(s), the industry and trends, your competition, and some marketing strategies. In Chapter 4, you will learn that the marketing plan is a lot like the business plan. It requires additional research, some analytic thought, and strategic planning. The business plan is your business concept's organizational tool, and the marketing plan is your communication tool.

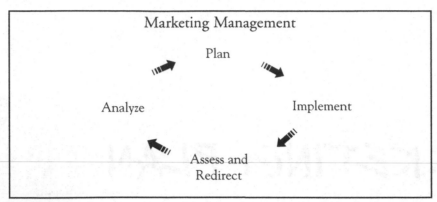

Figure 4-1. Marketing management.

There are four steps to the marketing plan:

Step 1: Analyze your market.

Step 2: Create a marketing plan.

Step 3: Implement your marketing plan.

Step 4: Assess and redirect your marketing strategies.

Creating a marketing plan, choosing a variety of marketing strategies, implementing creative marketing approaches, and re-evaluating the results is essential to increasing client, physician, payer, and community visibility, responsiveness, and referrals. Managing all of those activities is referred to as "marketing management" (Figure 4-1). Just like clinical management, marketing management strives to meet the rehab business concept's mission and organizational objectives.

Marketing and marketing management evolve around understanding the groups of variables that your rehab business will employ to influence the demand for your services or products. Conceptually, they are referred to as the "four P's": product, price, place, and promotion.[2] Over time, marketing experts have added a fifth P: position.

1. *Product (or service):* Any item or features of that item that is offered to the consumer for awareness or purchase.

2. *Price:* The cost of the service or product.

3. *Place:* Where and how you will provide access to your service or product.

4. *Promotion:* The communication of the benefits, price, and place of your service or product.

5. *Position:* How and where your service or product compares to your competitor's.

Product

Product (or service) has already been identified in earlier chapters. As you move ahead to Step 1, you will be asked to identify specific elements of your products and services that you will use to create marketing materials.

Price

The price of your services and products can be complicated, especially when third-party payers such as the federal and state governmental insurance funds are involved. There are several variables to keep in mind when deciding on your pricing. They include:

- Development and production costs, such as the time or software costs of creating an athlete's participation screening

- Fair market value, which is generally called "usual, customary, and realistic." Ask other professionals in your area what they are receiving for reimbursement from federal and state insurance programs, commercial insurers, workers' compensation, regional centers, and any other paying entity.

- Government regulations and fee schedules. Medicare fee rates, additions/deletions of codes, and other coding and billing tasks change frequently. Check with the Center for Medicare and Medicaid Services at www.cms.hhs.gov for the latest information.

- Third-party payer contracted fee schedules. When you call commercial insurers, ask them for a provider contract application and a fee schedule so you can see exactly how they want you to code and bill, and also how much you can expect to be paid, unless you negotiate a different payment rate.

- Other payer fee schedules and the client's ability to pay. Payers like the school system, regional systems, charities or foundations, and workers' compensation agencies all have different reimbursement rates. Also, consider the demographics of your present or potential client and their ability to pay either your cash price, the co-insurance, or non-billable services such as splints and other home management products.

- Local environment (competitor) pricing. Gather information about prices from nearby services or programs that are similar to yours (regardless if they are therapy-based or not) in order to see what area consumers are accustomed to paying. For example, if you are starting up an afterschool sensory program for autistic children, look at other area "Mommy and Me" or children's play and instructional classes and how much they cost. This is a good place to begin establishing your bottom dollar amount.

- Overhead expenses such as rent, licenses, permits, etc. In Chapter 6, you will learn how to fill out a start-up cost sheet, which will list all of the items you will need to know the costs of.

- Target market's budget and purchasing habits. Is your business situated in a low, medium, or high income area? You will need to price your services, products, and programs accordingly.

- Other business expenses such as payroll, taxes, etc.

Typically, the local market price for similar services and products and regional pricing by governmental funds (eg, the Medicare Physician Fee Schedule [www.cms.hhs.gov]) are the go-to benchmarks to begin strategizing on pricing. If you have a contract with payer entities, make sure to ask for their contracted fee schedule. Networking with other colleagues in your local area is also helpful. If you have hired a medical billing company, be sure to discuss and understand the pricing of your services and products. There are stiff penalties for violating federal guidelines and network contracted fees and billing guidelines. If your medical billing company fails to comply, you are still held accountable.

Place

Place can be where your rehab business is located, such as in a clinic setting. It also implies any other marketing activity where your target markets can receive access to your products and services. For example, you provide contracted adult mental health community life skills outreach programs in various community centers (place) and also provide van transportation (place) for those who need assistance.

Promotion

Promotion includes creating and communicating specific variables of your business, products, or services to your three different target markets that will increase their awareness or educate and persuade them to utilize and purchase the products or services that meet their particular needs. This is accomplished through different types of marketing strategies, such as networking or advertising. You were asked to select some marketing strategies to complete your business plan. You will learn more in Step 2.

Position

Position is the process of determining how well your rehab business is performing compared to your competitors, and how well you are increasing awareness and business from your clients and referral sources. Elements of positioning can be utilized as outcome measurements when addressing how successful your marketing strategies are meeting your goals. For example, your rehab business was mentioned in a local newspaper for providing a much-needed driving program for older adults that you personally marketed by speaking to area assisted-living centers and handing out small labeled key chains. You later received phone calls from potential clients because you marketed your unique service with a fun promotion.

STEP 1: ANALYZE YOUR MARKET

The bottom line is you have to have clients to stay in business. Furthermore, you may have to have a referral to evaluate and treat the client depending on your state's practice act. In addition, you may want or need to have a contract with a payer entity so you can get paid, which will require you to apply or qualify with the paying entity.

All of these statements have something in common—they explain your market. The market is "the set of all actual and potential buyers of a product or service."[2] There are four areas of the market that need to be analyzed to develop your marketing plan. This process is called "market analysis."

The four areas of market analysis include:
1. Review of the industry and emerging trends
2. Determine your target markets
3. Identify your competitors
4. Perform a product and service assessment

✛ Review of the Industry and Emerging Trends

In Chapter 3, you researched and made conclusions about your industry and emerging trends. You also considered various external and internal factors that impact your industry and your rehab business concept's ability to develop and sustain the necessary relationships between you and your target markets. In the global business world of marketing, the external impact factors are called the "macroenvironment" and the internal factors are considered the "microenvironment." Together, they are called the "marketing environment."[2] Effective and successful marketing is dependent on continuously watching and adapting to your marketing environment. As a review, complete the following exercises:

- What are some important social and economical factors affecting your market (eg, location, consumer characteristics, educational levels, income, buying habits, referral sources, competition, technology)?

  _____
  _____
  _____

- What are some of the legal factors affecting your market (eg, standards of practice, licensure or certification requirements, regulations, qualifications, competencies)?

  _____
  _____
  _____

- What are some of the local, state, and federal governmental factors affecting your market (eg, Medicare qualifications, HIPAA Privacy Standards, health care budget cuts, professional infringement)?

  _____
  _____
  _____

✛ Determine Your Target Markets

The rehab market in health care can be divided into three categories[3]:
1. Clients and potential clients
2. Referral sources
3. Payers

Each of those categories contains many types of smaller, specific markets with common characteristics and needs that are measurable and that your rehab business wants to influence. These are called the "target markets."

- Write down your target market (client) that you identified in your Business Plan (eg, clients with sports injuries or clients with hand injuries).

  _____

Marketing to clients or potential clients is the main thrust of your marketing plan. However, the decision to utilize your rehab business services or products, especially in health care, is usually dependent on needing a referral and the ability to pay either through a payer system or cash. Your marketing plan needs to address all three target markets involved in the client's decision process to be successful.

Referring to the three main health care target markets, list all of the target markets that you will need to market your rehab business services and products, too.

1. Clients/potential clients (eg, adolescent orthopedics):

    _____

    _____

    _____

    Write a typical profile (characteristics, needs) of your target market:

    _____

    _____

    _____

2. Referral sources (eg, high school coach):

    _____

    _____

    _____

    Write a typical profile (needs, demands) of your referral source:

    _____

    _____

    _____

3. Payers (eg, private pay):

    _____

    _____

    _____

    Write a typical profile (qualification requests, regulations) of your payer:

    _____

    _____

    _____

The various target markets you identified share the common characteristic of requiring knowledge of what your services and products include and achieve in order to decide whether they would recommend, purchase, or use them. You, on the other hand, need to recognize that there are certain elements that go into the informed decision process. Customers want the "five F's"[1]:

1. Function
2. Finances
3. Freedom
4. Feelings
5. Future

Your target markets want to know how your product or service will meet their particular need, how much and how reasonable your product or service is, how convenient and accessible it is, how it will affect or relate to their personal situation, and if purchasing or utilizing your product or service will have a positive effect on some aspect of their life. This client-centered concept should sound familiar to rehab business owners: educate the physician about your services, evaluate the referred client, establish professional rapport through compassion and communication, promote client-centered functional goals through your services and products, and provide measurable outcomes. Likewise, your referral and payer target markets also want to be educated, attended to, and personally communicated with in a manner to meet their needs and wants. Keeping mindful of the five F's will be vital in establishing your marketing strategies.

Continually ask yourself this question:

*   What function, freedom, and feelings about the future will your services and products provide to your potential clients, referral sources, and payers?

    _____

    _____

Example of Target Markets

Target Markets

Clients/Potential Clients	Referral Sources	Payers
Orthopedic injuries	Physicians	Managed care
Neurological disorders	Home health agencies	Organizations
Hand injuries	Case manager	Workers' compensation
Seniors	Adult children	Medicare
Pediatrics	School system	State funds
Athletes	Friends/family	Cash
Mentally challenged	Professionals	Insurance plans
High-risk adolescents	Chamber of commerce	Charities
Corporations	Churches	Private donation
High schools	Provider networks	Legal sponsors
Area businesses	Legal system	Trust funds
Injured workers	Insurance	Federal grants
Persons with chronic diseases	Alternative practitioners	Private grants
Spas	Office staff	Private parties
Low vision populations	Department of Motor Vehicles	Local government
Assisted-living centers	Clinical manager	Member network
Community centers	Business owner	Foundations

✛ Identify Your Competitors

Sound familiar? You completed the Competition Survey Chart in Chapter 3 (see p. 59) and identified your primary and secondary competitors of your rehab business. Complete the review statements below.

- Who is your primary competitor?_____
- What are their products and services? _____
- What are their marketing strategies? _____
- Who is your secondary competitor? _____
- What are their products and services? _____
- What are their marketing strategies? _____
- List the strengths/weaknesses of your rehab business compared to your competition (eg, location, price, reputation, personnel, experience, referrals, etc).

Strengths: Weaknesses:

1. _____   1. _____
2. _____   2. _____
3. _____   3. _____
4. _____   4. _____

✛ *Perform a Product and Service Assessment*

You need to readily describe the features, benefits, or advantages of your services or products to facilitate target market awareness, promotion (referral), and purchasing. Remember that your goal is to satisfy the "five F's" of customer wants.

- Write a description of each of your product or services (include what it does; specific goals it meets; features; benefits; how it works; when, where, and why someone would need it; and what is the emotional value of it).

  _____

  _____

  _____

- What advantages do your products or services have over your competition?

  _____

  _____

  _____

- What disadvantages are there?

  _____

  _____

  _____

This information will be used in formulating your marketing materials such as brochures, advertisements, or flyers.

Special Considerations for the Rehab Professional

If you are already a rehab business owner, perform an organizational assessment. The organizational assessment is an organization's reevaluation of its effectiveness relative to the patient population, the community, and the health care system itself.[3] Like the market analysis you just performed, you closely examine your external and internal factors. The external factors are similar to the market analysis, except, instead of addressing the possibilities, you identify the current external business issues and future impact factors. The internal factors are your daily business operations. Include everything from existing clients to medical records. Complete the Organizational Assessment on the next page.

Perform the SWOT Analysis to analyze how effectively your business is presently marketing to your existing clients and your other target markets. Items under the weakness category usually signify areas that are affecting your ability to attract and sustain your client and referral base. That is where your marketing plan efforts start first. It may be that your marketing strategies, such as brochures and networking with physicians, is adequate—a strength—but poor customer service or the lack of clinic parking prevents your marketing from being successful and, therefore, has become your weakness or threat for business success.

STEP 2: CREATE A MARKETING PLAN

A marketing plan is a tool to coordinate and implement information about the marketing objectives and strategies of the rehab business to meet the organizational and financial goals. Basically, you create a message that you deliver to your target markets by using marketing strategies to persuade them to buy or utilize your services or products.

✛ *Contents of a Marketing Plan*

Formally, the marketing plan takes on the look of a business plan. It contains several of the same elements, which include:
- Business description
- Business goals
- Description of products and services
- Industry description
- Strengths and obstacles
- Target market(s)

Organizational Assessment

External Factors		Internal Factors	
Rate: S (Strength) or W (Weakness)		Rate: O (Opportunities) or T (Threats)	
Competition:	_____	Operations:	_____
Regulations:	_____	Productivity:	_____
Current customers:	_____	Personnel development:	_____
Legal compliance:	_____	Reputation:	_____
Reimbursement:	_____	Customer service:	_____
Emerging trends:	_____	Financial management:	_____
Federal policies:	_____	Quality of care:	_____
Technology advances:	_____	Sales and marketing:	_____
Economic environment:	_____	Profitability:	_____

- Marketing strategies
- Implementation
- Assess and redirect

✛ Marketing Strategies

Remember the five P's? Product, price, place, promotion, and position are the fun, creative variables that affect the selection of information that becomes your message on the marketing materials you create. You have already identified your product or services, price, place, and position.

Promotions, promotional strategies, or selling tactics is what is commonly thought of as marketing. However, as you now know, it is only one element of marketing, and it is the showpiece. Promotional campaigns involve several different types of promotional materials specifically selected to tell your target markets the what, when, where, how, and sometimes how much of the features and benefits of your products and services. The image and message demonstrated by information contained on your promotional materials should be clear, simple, truthful, and value-centered (see Appendix C for examples of marketing materials).

Marketing strategies are divided into four categories:
1. Advertising
2. Sales promotion
3. Public relations
4. Personal selling

Advertising

Advertising is any paid form of written promotion of your products or services. Business cards, brochures, and ad placement in local newspapers are examples of advertising. Check with federal and state laws and professional associations since they may regulate certain advertising formats and language usage.

Sales Promotion

Sales promotions are marketing promotional incentives such as labeled water bottles or ink pens with your company's name or logo on them. Check with an attorney before offering free screenings or assessments at activities outside of your business location for liability purposes (eg, participating in a health fair and offering muscle testing). Also, keep in mind that anti-kickback laws prevent you from outright marketing to referral sources for the purpose of receiving something in exchange, such as referred clients. Your sales promotions need to be under $300.00 annually to all referral sources and equally available to all of your target markets.

Public Relations

Public relations are promotions centered around creating an image about your rehab business by performing charitable, humanitarian deeds such as volunteering to raise money for a local charity by cosponsoring a 5K race or networking by joining the local chamber of commerce. Your goal should be honorable and made in the context of your target markets.

Personal Selling

Personal selling is a promotional strategy that is performed regularly by you everyday and has minimal costs. The goal of personal selling is to build rapport and relationships with your target markets and your community. It includes networking, educating physicians and referral sources about your business, and all face-to-face communications. Joining the local chamber of commerce and speaking to schools, church groups, and other area businesses is a great way to increase awareness and promote your products and services.

Keep in mind that selecting which marketing strategies to implement in your marketing plan depends on several factors (see the next page for examples of marketing strategies):

- Specific needs of target market
- Your strengths and advantages over your competitors
- The amount of time and money budgeted for marketing
- State regulation limitations such as trademark usage (AOTA, APTA) or other slogans or words that are trademarked or copyrighted.

The marketing strategy component of the Marketing Plan Worksheet includes identifying the unique advantages or benefits of your products and services that will be highlighted on your marketing materials. Revisit your product and service assessment in Step 1, and keep the five F's of consumer wants in mind. Generally, the prices for health care services are not specified on the marketing materials, especially if you are getting paid by third-party payers. However, stating the price for other services such as the costs for an 8-week yoga program for osteoporosis is appropriate and even vital for the client's decision process on whether to attend your program or your competitor's program.

Additionally, the marketing strategy component asks you to specify general guidelines for customer service. The importance of customer service is often overlooked and underrated. The first impression is a lasting impression and requires attention to satisfying your target market's needs and wants with accurate information, politeness, and constant follow-up conversation. Identify the exact rules of engagement that will be followed by everyone involved in promoting your business. Keep those posted as informative reminders.

Tips and Tools

There are several resources available for purchasing or creating your own marketing materials:

Promotional Materials Companies:
- www.bestimpressions.com
- www.nebs.com

Marketing Software:
- Marketing Plan Pro 2003 (www.mplans.com)

- www.orientaltrading.com
- www.baudville.com
- www.4imprint.com
- OfficeReady Marketing Plans (www.templatezone.com)
- Plan Write Marketing Planner (www.planware.org)

Collect marketing materials from area businesses, cut out advertisements from trade newspapers and magazines, and take notice of the marketing materials that catch your attention. Use these examples to assist in formulating your marketing materials. You are going to use your business name, domain names, or variations of those to put on your marketing materials. Copyright and trademark your business names, logos, slogans, or phrases when necessary.

Marketing Strategies

Advertising

- Ads
- Brochures
- Flyers
- Direct mail
- Business cards
- Prescription pads
- Booklets
- Calendars
- Promotional gifts
- Telemarketing
- Email postcards
- Fax broadcasting
- Postcards
- Newsletters
- Inserts
- TV
- Radio
- Internet
- Posters

Personal Selling

- Thank you cards
- Birthday cards
- Ask for referrals
- Lunch/meet with your referrals
- Seasonal greetings/gifts
- Treats/promotional gifts
- Leave articles on table
- Message board
- Referral board
- Picture board
- Gift certificates
- Business cards
- Flyers
- Brochures
- Networking
- Volunteer
- Resource
- Web site
- Email address
- Cell phone/pager
- Fax
- Mailing/billing inserts

Public Relations

- News releases
- Study or survey
- Case studies
- Article writing
- Letter to the editor
- Column writing
- Testimonials
- Guest lectures
- Seminars
- Health fair
- Volunteering
- Media kit mailings
- Join associations
- Join networking groups
- Focus groups
- Host meetings/seminars
- Lunch and learns
- Open house
- Power breakfasts
- Happy hour
- TV/radio guests
- Involvement in community
- Form alliances
- Donate to charity
- Donate to fundraisers

Sales Promotion

- Patient referral incentives
- Open house
- Sweepstakes
- Office giveaways
- Free assessments
- Discounts
- Coupons
- Gift certificates
- Free demonstrations
- Free samples
- Phone hold messaging
- Treats at your reception window
- Holiday goodies
- Trade show giveaways

Marketing Plan Worksheet

Business name: _____

Company description: _____
_____

Mission statement: _____

Vision statement: _____

Business goals:

      A. 6 to 12 months: _____

      B. 12 to 24 months: _____

      C. 24 to 60 months: _____

Description of products/services: _____

Industry description and trends:_____

Possible market obstacles to overcome:

      A. Industry: _____

      B. Target markets: _____

      C. Competition: _____

      D. Products/services: _____

Strengths/opportunities our company, products, and services have in market:

      A. External: _____

      B. Internal: _____

Target market needs and wants: _____

Target Market(s)

A.   To whom will we be selling or promoting our products/services?

      1. _____

      2. _____

      3. _____

      4. _____

B.   How will we target our consumer?

      1. _____

      2. _____

      3. _____

      4. _____

C.   Where will we sell/promote ("place" or area)?

      1. _____

      2. _____

      3. _____

      4. _____

D.   What is the product/service we are marketing?

      1. _____

      2. _____

      3. _____

      4. _____

E.   How much will our target market spend on our product/service?

      $_____ per unit, hour, month, or year

(continued)

Marketing Strategies

A. List the features (advantages, benefits) of your product/service:

1. _____

2. _____

3. _____

4. _____

B. Estimate how much your product/service will cost:

1. To develop and produce: _____

2. Fair market value: _____

3. Fee options (flexibility): _____

4. Sales/taxes: _____

5. To maintain customer service: _____

6. Third-party payer rates: _____

7. How much our competition charges: _____

8. Rates: _____   *Profit margin* gain: _____ %

C. Specify general guidelines for customer service:

1. _____

2. _____

3. _____

4. _____

5. _____

D. Image:

1. Company name:_____

2. Company logo (name, colors, tag lines):_____

E. Attach copies of your business card, logo, or other slogans here:

(Example)

Jacksonville's

Orthopedic

Group

Come for the healing!
Stay for the caring!

Location   Email
Phone   Web site

Logo: trademark, copyright, registered, etc.   Slogan:

Come for the healing!
Stay for the caring!

(continued)

Marketing Plan Booklet © Ultimate Rehab, LLC 2001

Marketing Action Plan

A. Identify marketing budget:

Time: _____

Money: _____

B. Identify promotion types:

Promotion:	Cost:	Time:	Target Market:
1. _____	_____	_____	_____
2. _____	_____	_____	_____
3. _____	_____	_____	_____
4. _____	_____	_____	_____
5. _____	_____	_____	_____
6. _____	_____	_____	_____
7. _____	_____	_____	_____
8. _____	_____	_____	_____
9. _____	_____	_____	_____

C. Establish a time line: 18 months (Put letter next to promotional type above)

- D: Daily
- W: Weekly
- M: Monthly
- Q: Quarterly
- B: Bi-annually
- A: Annually

D. Determine your marketing goals:

1. _____

2. _____

3. _____

E. Who is going to perform the marketing activities: _____

Assess and Redirect

A. There is an increase in the number of clients per week. Percentage: _____ %

B. There is an increase in overall gross business revenue. Percentage: _____ %

C. We conducted a client survey on how they heard about us.   ❏ Yes   ❏ No

D. Which marketing promotional types were the most effective? _____

E. Which marketing promotional types were the least effective? _____

F. What was the ratio on return? (number of dollars spent on increase in revenue?)_____

G. Have you created greater visibility and business than your competitors?_____

D. Measure the success/failures of your goals.

1. Did you meet your goals?_____

2. If yes, establish an ongoing action plan. _____

3. If no, redirect your marketing effort with new choices of promotional types or re-evaluate what your target audience wants and needs based on client, referral, and payer surveys. List new choices.

_____

_____

_____

_____

STEP 3: IMPLEMENT YOUR MARKETING PLAN

Now it's time to put your marketing strategies and promotional materials to work. Implementing your marketing plan requires you to perform five actions:
1.   Appoint someone to manage the marketing plan and process.
2.   Identify a marketing plan budget.
3.   Identify which promotional strategies will be employed.
4.   Create a marketing plan time line.
5.   Establish marketing plan goals.

Use the Marketing Plan Worksheet (pp. 87–89) as your marketing management guide. Set measurable, definable, reachable, and sizable goals that can be evaluated in timed intervals such as every 3 or 6 months. For example, you want to increase your number of clients per week by 10% in 3 months or you will personally host free lunch-and-learn seminars at area community centers and obtain three new referral sources in 6 months. Marketing experts suggest nine marketing attempts in 18 months to establish a successful marketing plan.[4] Keep in mind that the promotional strategy choices need to meet a specific target market's needs and wants. Revisit your target market profiles to assist you.

STEP 4: ASSESS AND REDIRECT YOUR MARKETING STRATEGIES

In health care, outcome measurements allow the rehab professional to systemically determine what, which, where, when, and why a particular set of clinical treatment practice standards produced the results. Likewise, evaluating your marketing plan is necessary to avoid spending time and money on operational activities that reap no rewards and do not accomplish any goals. Typically, your marketing goals are to increase the number of clients per day or week, which, in turn, increases your revenue. However, it is important to consistently increase your referral sources and payers to obtain long-term business and financial success.

An example of assessments and redirect marketing tasks is given in the marketing plan worksheet. Create the assessment markers that will measure the success or failure of the five action steps of your marketing action plan specific to your marketing goals within all three target market categories. If you are unable to identify why certain marketing strategies did not work, go straight back to the target market for which they were selected and ask for feedback. Many times, we assume the answers instead of actively finding the solutions.

Special Considerations for the Rehab Professional

Here are some general guidelines to keep in mind when marketing to the various target markets.

Clients

*   The easiest way to find out what your clients and potential clients want and will pay for is conducting a client survey. Create a survey that asks specific questions in regard to the five P's: products (and services), price, place, promotion, and position. Utilize the survey information to develop your marketing strategies, action plan, and redirection plan.

Referral Sources

*   The same holds true for referral sources. Although not as easy and comfortable to do, your referral sources are vital to your business survival. Keep in mind that physicians are just like you—busy, but wanting to attract clients also. Create a referral survey that is short, clear, and direct. For example, what types of services do your clients need (eg, balance program or water therapy, etc)? Ask questions with checklist answers so the time needed to complete the survey is minimal. Educate the referral sources by writing your business name, mission and vision statements, and your business goals strategically on the survey. Be ready to hand the referral source a thank you note or business card with your contact and location information on it. Even better, leave behind prescription pads with your business name, services and products, contact information, types of payments available, and a map on the back.

Payers

- Contract managers of third-party payers will typically ask for your business information, such as location, products and services offered, staff license numbers, and types of equipment.[5] If you are negotiating a contract, be ready to support your pricing for your services and products by conducting a local fee survey of competitive rates. Payers, like clients and referral sources, want to know why they should have a contract with your business and whether you offer unique services. Niche programs such as aquatic services or wellness programs are a plus. Be sure to have your marketing materials ready to send to your payers before you contact them. Follow up with phone calls, mailing, and ongoing conversations to establish a rapport of positive communication and image. You may also want to include letters from former clients or referrals to support your high standards of care, unique services, and client accessibility.

Remember, marketing means telling your target markets what they get, not what you do. If you need additional assistance in completing and implementing a marketing plan, contact SCORE, "Counselors to America's Small Business" (www.score.org) or a health care or marketing consultant.

CHAPTER 4 SUMMARY

Developing your marketing plan involves choosing a variety of marketing strategies, implementing creative marketing approaches, and re-evaluating the results. These are essential to increasing client, physician, payer, and community visibility, responsiveness, and referrals.

Step 1: Analyze Your Market
- Who are your target market(s)?
  - o Clients or potential clients:

  _____

  _____

  - o Referral sources:

  _____

  _____

  - o Payers:

  _____

  _____

Step 2: Create a Marketing Plan
- What marketing strategies will best communicate your business's benefits, advantages, and goals?

  _____

  _____

  _____

- Which marketing strategies will you utilize for each target market?

  _____

  _____

  _____

Step 3: Implement Your Marketing Plan
- What is your marketing budget?_____
- What are your three main marketing goals?
  - ❏ Increase referral sources.
  - ❏ Increase patient volume.
  - ❏ Increase awareness of our services.
  - ❏ Obtain a payer contract.
  - ❏ Obtain additional funding.
  - ❏ Obtain more staffing.
  - ❏ Promote advocacy or education.
  - ❏ Other:_____
- Who will perform the marketing activities and follow up? _____

Step 4: Assess and Redirect Your Marketing Strategies
- Are your marketing plan objectives specific, measurable, and attainable?
  - ❏ Yes   ❏ No, I need to redirect my strategies.

Action Plan
  - ❏ Complete the marketing plan.
  - ❏ Revisit your business plan to update or confirm any marketing information that was gathered previously. If you received outside funds to operate your rehab business, make sure your financials in the business plan match your marketing plan budget. Marketing plan goals and how you achieve them will also be very important to the lending institutions.

REFERENCES

1. Abrams R. *The Successful Business Plan: Secrets and Strategies*. Palo Alto, CA: Running 'R' Media; 2000:9-11.

2. Kotler P, Armstrong G. *Marketing: An Introduction*. 5th ed. Upper Saddle River, NJ: Prentice Hall; 2000.

3. Richmond T. Marketing. In: McCormack G, Jaffe E, Goodman-Lavey M, eds. *The Occupational Therapy Manager*. 4th ed. Bethesda, MD: American Occupational Therapy Association; 2003:177-192.

4. Kremer J, McComas JD. *High Impact Marketing on a Low-Impact Budget*. Rocklin, CA: Prima Publishing; 1997.

5. Le Postollec M. Making your business attractive to HMOs. *Advance for Physical Therapists and PT Assistants* [serial online]. 2000;11(14):34. Available at: http://physical-therapy.advanceweb.com/Editorial/Search/AViewer.aspx?AN=PT_p34.html&AD=07-10-2000. Accessed October 29, 2008.

SUGGESTED READING

Burrus D. Online advertising. *Advance for Directors in Rehabilitation* [serial online]. 2007. Available at: http://rehabilitation-director.advanceweb.com/Editorial/Content/Editorial.aspx?CC=101525. Accessed January 26, 2009.

Glinn J. Marketing strategies for small practices. *Advance for Physical Therapists and PT Assistants*. 2001;12(11):9-10.

Kelley J. Market strategy: build relationships through marketing and ensure your survival. *Advance for Directors in Rehabilitation* [serial online]. 2001;10(1):16. Available at: http://rehabilitation-director.advanceweb.com/Editorial/Search/AViewer.aspx?AN=DR_p16.html&AD=01-01-2001. Accessed October 29, 2008.

Kelley J. Spread the news: market your outcomes to physicians, payers, and patients. *Advance for Directors in Rehabilitation* [serial online]. 2001;10(7):14. Available at: http://rehabilitation-director.advanceweb.com/Editorial/Search/AViewer.aspx?AN=DR_p14.html&AD=07-01-2001. Accessed October 29, 2008.

Kintler D, Adams B. *Independent Consulting: Your Comprehensive Guide to Building Your Own Consulting Business*. Holbrook, MA: Adams Media Corp; 1998.

LaRue S. Standing apart: examining the link between meeting patients' needs and marketing. *Advance for Directors in Rehabilitation* [serial online]. 2007;16(7):18 Available at: http://rehabilitation-director.advanceweb.com/Editorial/Search/AViewer.aspx?AN=DR_07jul1_drp18.html&AD=07-01-2007. Accessed October 29, 2008.

Le Postollec M. Blueprint for success: marketing are the keys to a successful program. *Advance for Physical Therapists and PT Assistants* [serial online]. 2001;12(9):8. Available at: http://physical-therapy.advanceweb.com/Editorial/Search/AViewer.aspx?AN=PT_01may7_ptp8.html&AD=05-07-2001. Accessed October 30, 2008.

Levinson J, Levinson J. Here's the plan: 5 minutes is all you need to create a top-notch marketing plan—and get your business ready for success. *Entrepreneur*. Feb 2008:92-97.

Levinson J, Levinson J. Startup Guide to Guerrilla Marketing: A Simple Battle Plan for First-Time Marketers. Entrepreneur Press. 2008.

Martin P. Direct access: eight steps can lead to better marketing. *Advance for Directors in Rehabilitation* [serial online]. 2001;10(6):13-15. Available at: http://rehabilitation-director.advanceweb.com/Editorial/Search/AViewer.aspx?AN=DR_p13.html&AD=06-01-2001. Accessed October 30, 2008.

McPherson D. Putting your practice in the spotlight. *Advance for Occupational Therapy Practitioners* [serial online]. Available at: http://occupational-therapy.advanceweb.com/Editorial/Search/AViewer.aspx?AN=OT_cover.html&AD=02-28-2000. Accessed October 30, 2008.

Pinson L, Jinnett J. *Steps to Small Business Start-Up*. 4th ed. Chicago, IL: Dearborn; 2000.

Small Business Administration. Market and price. Available at: http://www.sba.gov/smallbusinessplanner/manage/marketandprice/index.html. Accessed December 30, 2008.

Turner C. Rehab marketing. *Rehab Management* [serial online]. Feb/March 2000. Available at: http://www.rehabpub.com/rehabec/232000/5.asp. Accessed March 26, 2003.

ELECTRONIC RESOURCES

www.logobee.com: Online logo design and web design company.

IMPLEMENTATION

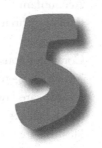

Dave Powers, PT, DPT, MA, MBA

Tammy Richmond, MS, OTRL

CHAPTER OBJECTIVES

✔ Gather advice and consultation from experts.
✔ Complete your operational infrastructure.
✔ Build your management skills and standards of care.
✔ Promote professional competency and code of ethics.

It's time to put your business plan to work! You have your "roadmap" to direct you toward implementing a successful rehab business. Now, it is all about action. This chapter will present a general template of administrative, managerial, and operational tasks that will assist you in accomplishing your business plan objectives. In addition, you will learn the concept of evidence-based management and professional competency—all of which impact your ability to implement the best standards of practice.

Many of these tasks happen all at once and can fall into any order that works best for your situation. Several of the implementation tools suggested can be found in Appendices D through G. Implementation of your rehab business is divided into four main steps:

Step 1: Gather advice and consultation from experts.
Step 2: Complete your operational infrastructure.
Step 3: Build your management skills and standards of care.
Step 4: Promote professional competency and code of ethics.

STEP 1: GATHER ADVICE AND CONSULTATION FROM EXPERTS

It is important to obtain advice and services from individuals who are experts in their fields to assist in the details of business and health care operations and compliance, therefore limiting unnecessary risks and common business mistakes.

Consider consulting with or hiring the following experts:
- Accountant
- Banker or financial advisor
- Colleagues
- Computer consultant
- Insurance agent
- Health care lawyer
- Small business consultant
- Health care consultant
- Professional organization (state and national associations)
- Space planner
- Suppliers
- Web designer
- Advisory positions such as board of directors, advisory committee
- Professional peers such as those you could find by belonging to the special interest sections of your professional organizations

If you are buying, selling, or considering to become a business partner to an already existing business practice, then a practice analysis needs to be performed and presented to you, including specific financial statements and other supportive documents. See Appendix D for a checklist of "Buying or Selling a Practice."

If you are mainly interested in expanding your present operations to new programs or services, start first by speaking with various experts from the list above that will clarify the business opportunities or any restrictions to actual program expansion and new services. You will also need to include key conversations with your payers, your referral sources (if applicable), and any person you will be reporting to in order to make sure operational vision and mission is understood and aligned with overall business goals and not just human interest. Next, go back to Chapter 1 and complete the Market Research Checklist and the SWOT analysis on a list of program ideas you have generated. This task should begin to eliminate or identify the feasible ideas. Then, review the market research checklist again and complete all of the questions with details. Write your business plan with these details just like you would with a new business idea. Create internal and external operational strategic tasks to finalize your program or service expansion. For example: internally, create a client survey asking about their interests both in new services and their ability to pay or participate, and schedule brainstorming sessions with your staff to flush out details and examine validity; externally, meet with potential target markets such as potential client types or the referral sources and survey their needs and expectations.

Overall, your goal is to demonstrate program or service validity and feasibility to reduce the risks inherent with all new business ideas or idea expansions. Your implementation of your program expansion follows the remaining parts of this chapter. If your program is a nonprofit business structure, your business plan will act as the support materials to complete the necessary IRS documentation requirements, and your implementation and financial management will support the parameters of not-for-profit organizational goals as provided by the donor, grant, foundation, and other charitable entities you are working for.

STEP 2: COMPLETE YOUR OPERATIONAL INFRASTRUCTURE

Your operational infrastructure will consist of creating various manuals and documents and performing multiple business and health care tasks. They can be divided into five main categories:
- Small business start-up tasks
- Clinical documentation
- Systems documentation
- Workflow management
- Facility management

Start-Up Tasks Checklist

- ❐ File partnership, corporation, or LLC papers with the Secretary of State's office.
- ❐ Complete any necessary legal contracts or agreements.
- ❐ Register business names and the domain name.
- ❐ Register copyrights and trademarks.
- ❐ Choose a location for the business.*
- ❐ Check zoning laws and obtain permits and licenses.
- ❐ Check work space for ADA requirements and compliance.
- ❐ File state tax forms with the Franchise Tax Board.
- ❐ Contact the IRS for information regarding federal tax schedules.
- ❐ Apply for a *state sales tax number.*
- ❐ Apply for a federal employee identification number if you have employees.
- ❐ Apply for a *tax identification number.*
- ❐ Obtain workers' compensation insurance, if applicable.
- ❐ Order any required public notices.
- ❐ Obtain business insurance.*
- ❐ Set up an accounting system.
- ❐ Open a business checking account.
- ❐ Print marketing materials.
- ❐ Purchase equipment and supplies.*
- ❐ Order inventory, signage, and fixtures.
- ❐ Set up your Web site.
- ❐ Join associations and local memberships.
- ❐ File quarterly and annual compliance reports such as tax filings, employee withholding, business structure reports, workers' compensation, and labor laws.

* See Appendix D.

✚ Small Business Start-Up Tasks

Use the Start-Up Tasks Checklist above in completing typical small business activities. Federal and state policies and legislative changes occur frequently, so some of these tasks may or may not apply specifically to your rehab business. Small business legal counsel is highly recommended. Remember, many of these tasks require specific turnaround time and processing, so manage your schedule accordingly (see Appendix D).

✚ Clinical Documentation

To implement the daily operations of your new business, you will need to have a number of health care components in place. Many of these components are required by federal and state health care laws and regulations, or are required to comply with the standards of practice within the rehab community. This chapter includes those components that are most important for health care compliance. There are many other health care and management tasks that are necessary for business success that will not be covered. Consult with management books specific to your industry for guidance and learning.

An adequate and properly written record of evaluation, intervention, and outcomes of provided services is necessary at so many levels within the health care practice daily operations. Over time, it has become the most important tool of communication, compliance, and reimbursement. There are two main components to clinical documentation:

1. Medical record
2. Coding and billing

The purpose of clinical documentation is both legal and professional for the following reasons[1]:
- It act as client's legal record of medical care.
- It articulates the rationale for provision of therapy services and the relationship of this service to the client's outcomes.
- It reflects the therapist's clinical reasoning and professional judgment.
- It creates a chronological record of client status, occupational therapy services provided to the client, and client outcomes.
- It is a tool for quality improvement audits.
- It is a means for determining reimbursement.
- It is a source of data to demonstrate compliance.
- It is a tool for collecting data for research.

The medical record is documentation to provide a chronological record of the client's condition and the appropriateness, effectiveness, and necessity of interventions, and to facilitate a client-centered approach to the overall therapy sessions.

There are five necessary clinical documentation types:
1. Evaluation
2. Treatment plan or plan of care (POC)
3. Encounter note or treatment note
4. Progress note
5. Discharge summary

First, the evaluation is data gathered through standardized or non-standardized assessments of the client's functional performance. If your business model is nonprofit, your assessment may be based on what the grant or donation entity requires or expects you to report.

For insurance purposes, the expected items of an evaluation are the following:
- Name
- Date of birth
- Client's gender
- Referring physician
- Onset date of injury or illness
- Start of care date
- Medical diagnosis and ICD 9 codes
- Precautions and contraindications
- Specific problem areas evaluated; measurements
- Interventions; frequency, intensity, duration
- Plan of care (short-term goals and long-term goals)

Make sure the evaluation contains a medical history to support the plan of care and prior level of function. Scores of standardized testing should be presented without interpretation of its meaning to the client. Basically, the evaluation should be based on objective information and not subjective opinion.

Second, the treatment plan or plan of care (POC) documents the necessity of therapy, identifies the procedures, modalities, frequency, and duration, and it addresses functional (occupational) performance areas. Goals must be reasonable, realistic, and time-limited, and they should include the potential for returning the client to his or her prior functional status. The best standards of practice require that we identify and utilize outcome measurements. There is no one standard of an outcome measurement, but, universally, the client's pain level has been accepted as an outcome measurement. If you are billing insurance carriers or belong to a provider network (a membership organization that negotiates your third party payer contracts for you), they may require your practice to implement a specific outcome measurement tool (eg, the FOTO outcome measurement data tool).

Third, the treatment encounter note is your daily treatment note. It is usually written after each therapy intervention session. It should document the skilled treatment activities and modalities and how they relate to the client's functional roles or activities of daily living. Stay away from subjective writing. Instead, report objectively about the client's response to the therapy session. The signature of the treating therapist and total therapy time is required. You will use this encounter note to fill out the superbill with corresponding procedural codes in order to bill for services.

Next, the progress note is a type of clinical documentation that summarizes the intervention and provides the information to support the medical necessity of your services. Generally, it is written every time you observe a significant change in the client's function or response to your treatment. A progress note should be written every 10 treatment sessions, or at least once during a treatment interval (30 days) depending on your payer's requirements. Your progress note should identify any changes to the POC or change in your client's status and explain how your treatment is assisting the client toward reaching the short- or long-term functional goals. For purposes of billing insurance carriers, make sure you identify the body part and side of body you are treating, and specifically write your note to address the therapeutic intervention that you will assign a billing code to. For example, if you are working on balance, then you must address the objective content of your intervention and use words that correspond to the billing code definition of neuromuscular re-education. You will learn more in Chapter 6.

Lastly, the discharge summary acts as your overall objective summary to the client's entire treatment interval with you. Documentation must include details like the number of treatment sessions and any scores of standardized testing. In addition, you need to address whether the short- and long-term goals were met and the parameters of the home program of therapeutic exercises or activities you gave the client, then indicate any follow-up recommendations you have.

Your medical record needs to answer these overall questions[1]:

- What was the client's functional (occupational) performance level at the time of evaluation?
- What are the client's occupational goals?
- What interventions were provided?
- Were the goals met?
- Does the documentation show evidence that the client is improving in specific areas of performances?
- Does the documentation contain information that the client, client's family, or caregivers were involved in setting goals?
- Have you documented the reasons for any changes to the plan of care?
- Are the treatment methods consistent with goals?
- What was the client's functional or occupational performance at the end of treatment?

Coding and billing are necessary if you are billing third party payers such as insurance carriers for your services. Basics to learning how to bill for reimbursement will be addressed in Chapter 6.

Tips and Tools

It is important to know how to write short-term and long-term goals. There are four components to writing acceptable functional goals. They are:

1. *Performance*: what you want the client to do in an objective, measurable behavior. For example, "client will lift the 10 lb box with both upper extremities 3 times from the floor to the work table."

2. *Criteria*: what level of performance is needed to meet the outcome of the behavior. For example, "client will lift the 10 lb box with both upper extremities 3 times from the floor to the work table with proper body mechanics."

3. *Conditions*: the when, where, how, or under what circumstances the behavior will be modified by the skilled therapist or environment. For example, "client will lift the 10 lb box with both upper extremities 3 times from the floor to the work table with proper body mechanics and without verbal cueing from the therapist."

4. *Time Frame*: add the date the goal can be realistically met. For example, "client will lift the 10 lb box with both upper extremities 3 times from the floor to the work table with proper body mechanics and without verbal cueing from the therapist for 10 minutes in four sessions."

✛ *Systems Documentation*

The purpose of systems documentation is to internally promote and develop the goals and mission of the business, to promote employee development and human resource guidelines, and to externally act as a legal record of the organization's operations (both health care and small business activities).

There are two main categories of systems documentation:
1. Clinical documentation (that you just learned about)
2. Compliance documentation

Compliance documentation is written records that are required or recommended to comply with federal and state policies and regulations or which represent the best standards of practice. They include but are not limited to:

*   *Standards of practice*: therapy practice requirements of practitioners for the delivery of occupational or physical therapy services. They can be found through the corresponding national associations AOTA and APTA.

*   *Code of ethics*: public statement of the common set of values and principles used to promote and maintain high standards of behavior in occupational and physical therapy. They can be found through the corresponding national associations AOTA and APTA.

*   *Licensing or certification laws and regulations*: sets of rules and policies that govern rehab professionals established at the state government. You should obtain a copy for your personal records and understanding. Contact your state licensing or certification boards for application and renewal of your professional license or certifications.

*   *Supervisory Guidelines*: guidelines or regulations explaining the use of assistants and aides, supervision, client-related tasks, and limitations. They are available through the national and state associations and licensing or certification boards.

*   *HIPAA notice of privacy policy*: a statement given to patients to inform them of their privacy rights with respect to their personal health information (PHI). The notice must also be visibly posted in the practice. All personnel are required to be HIPAA trained and made aware of changes on a regular basis. Visit www.hhs.gov/ocr/hipaa/privacy.html for more information.

*   *Policy and procedure manual**: an operational tool that acts as a guidebook for practice management. Put your policies and procedures in writing. Communicate the policies and procedures to all of your employees. Have them sign a form stating that they have reviewed and understand all of the policies and procedures. Your staff must be informed of all updates to ensure that they are consistently applied and followed. You should review and update your policy and procedures annually. The main components typically found in a policy and procedure manual include:
    o   Clinic philosophy
    o   Administrative management
    o   Regulatory compliance
    o   Personnel
    o   Clinical care/interventions
    o   Documentation
    o   Facility management
    o   Fiscal management

*   *Informed consent**: a form that explains the treatment process and provides an avenue of communication to assist in risk management. Each patient, or his or her legal guardian, must sign a consent form. A copy must be given to the patient, and another kept in his or her medical record.

*   *Unusual occurrence report**: a report that is filled out by you or your staff any time there is an incident in your clinic. It is a confidential document that is to be used by you and your attorney. You are not to document in the medical record that one has been filled out.

*   *Medical records*: documentation needed to provide a chronological record of the client's condition and the appropriateness, effectiveness, and necessity of treatment interventions, and it is needed to facilitate a client-centered approach to plan of care. The following additional information should be found within the client's medical record:

---

* See Appendix D.

- ○ Client's name
- ○ Medical record number (if used)
- ○ Client's physician
- ○ Client's diagnosis
- ○ Client's past medical history
- ○ Client's current medical history
- ○ Client's precautions
- ○ Therapist objective evaluation
- ○ Assessment of patient's condition
- ○ Problems identified by patient and therapist
- ○ Treatment goals (short- and long-term)
- ○ Treatment plan
- ○ Rehab potential
- ○ Estimated time to achieve goals
- ○ Patient's understanding and agreement to treatment program

Outcome management/outcome measurements:
- Employee files (personnel files): A file must be kept on every employee hired into your organization. This information is confidential and should be kept in a safe and locked place. The file should include the following:
  - ○ Employee job description
  - ○ Employee agreement
  - ○ Copy of license, certification, advanced certifications, or credentials
  - ○ Copy of CPR card
  - ○ Employees' personnel information such as time records, vacations, etc
  - ○ Employee attendance
  - ○ Employee's continuing education records
  - ○ Employee's competency evaluations
  - ○ Performance evaluations
  - ○ Peer reviews
- Employee handbook: A small booklet containing information about benefits, time off, and more that comply with your state's labor laws and your company's policy and procedure manual.
- Any other required accreditation paperwork: If you belong to a provider network, they may require additional documentation such as patient satisfaction surveys, chart review tools, or risk management tools.
- Wages and benefits: There are many regulations that govern wages and benefits that serve to protect both the employee and the employer. This information is generally classified under the term "employment law." You will need to obtain advice and comply with wages and benefits regulations specific to your state and location. Here is some general information about rights and laws regarding wages and benefits[2]:
  - ○ The Fair Labor Standards Act (FLSA) requires employers to pay employees at least the hourly minimum wage plus overtime worked, except for exempt employees such as independent contractors or volunteers.
  - ○ Types of wages: minimum and subminimum wage (such as disabled workers).
  - ○ Workweek standards: employees must pay at least minimum wage for all regular workweek hours. Overtime wages depend on the type of employee.
  - ○ Employers must retain records of employees' earnings for 3 years.
  - ○ Employers are required to post labor posters: FLSA, The Family and Medical Leave Act, The Job Safety and Health Protection, The Equal Employment Opportunity, The Employee Polygraph Protection Act. An additional poster may include workers' compensation.
  - ○ Employment and self-employment taxes must be paid.
  - ○ Benefits plans include defined contribution plans, defined benefit plans, stock options plans, IRAs and Keoghs, vesting, and health insurance.

- Workplace safety: It is important to protect yourself, your employees, and your clients, and to comply with laws and regulations regarding work-related accidents or illnesses. Policies are established by the U.S. Department of Labor Occupational Safety and Health Association (OSHA). There are new recordkeeping rules and labor law posters that may be required in your business location. Check with your advisory experts.

Your operational infrastructure is the foundation for implementing your business plan goals and, most importantly, your health care practice activities. There are several ways to obtain documents, such as purchasing them through your national association's online store or through other publishing vendors like www.ultimaterehab.com. Use the Management and Operations Checklist on pp. 103-104 to assist you with performing all of the necessary operational activities that will make your practice comply and succeed. (Also found in Appendix D.)

Tips and Tools

Fraud and abuse is a major concern regarding Medicare and Medicaid programs. There are several governmental policies to know[5]:

- The False Claims Act: a civil law that targets the submission of false claims to federal health care programs and allows for financial recovery for each false claim. It also includes a provision for whistleblowers to share in the government's fraud recovery.

- The Anti-Kickback Statute: a criminal law that prohibits the payment of any money or other incentive to induce the referral or order of any service or item reimbursed by the Medicare and Medicaid programs.

- The Exclusion Authority: allows Health and Human Services to bar entities and individuals from participating directly or indirectly in federal health care programs.

- The Stark Law: a civil statute that prohibits payment by Medicare for certain types of services if the services were ordered by a physician who has a prohibited financial interest or compensation relationship with the entity that is billing for them. There are exceptions.

✛ Work Flow Management

Workflow management involves the operational tasks that are performed regularly that create an effective and efficient business and, therefore, increase productivity and profitability. Your daily workflow is personalized to your specific type of business structure and organization and management skills. The Workflow Management Checklist is an example of how to organize your practice management tasks (see p. 105).

✛ Facility Management

Operational tasks that often get left behind in the busyness of a new practice are those that could inadvertently cause you to fail. The Facility Management Checklist on p. 106 is a reminder list of items that should be checked regularly to avoid unnecessary liabilities or expensive repair needs (see Tips and Tools on p. 108).

Special Considerations for the Rehab Professional

Payment for your services or products requires that you have knowledge and skills in several reimbursement components. They include:

- Sources of payment: Public funds are available through federal and state insurance and grant programs, such as Medicare, Medicaid, workers' compensation, Individuals with Disabilities Education Act (IDEA), Social Services Block Grant program, Community Mental Health Centers Act, and others.[3] Private payment is available through insurance plans such as Blue Cross, managed care organizations, cash payments, and other private-paying entities. Each payment source may require specific billing forms and coding.

- Payment methodologies: The fee for service methodology is payment as a rate per unit of service based on a fee schedule using codes for each service provided. Prospective rate methodology is based on the average costs per specific type of illness or injury for a specific duration of time. Therefore, payment is restricted by national averages (eg, the Medicare RBRVS fee schedule). Capitation methodology pays the provider per health plan member per month regardless of service usage. Therefore, payment is usually lower (eg, HMOs).

Management and Operations Checklist

☐ Professional licenses and certifications renewals in personnel file

☐ Professional PDUs/CEUs completed and in personnel file

☐ Professional liability insurance for each therapist, practice

☐ General commercial insurance

☐ Workers' compensation insurance

☐ Business license renewal

☐ Yearly property taxes

☐ Quarterly federal tax return

☐ Quarterly contribution return (EDD)

☐ Quarterly wage and withholding report

☐ Secretary of State; Corporation fee

☐ Yearly corporation federal and state tax return

☐ Business checking account in name of business

☐ Accounting software for invoicing or billing

☐ Independent contractor agreements (if applicable)

☐ Job descriptions

☐ Business description

☐ Documentation requirements (Code of Ethics, Standards of Practice, Copy of Laws and Regulations, Practice Guidelines, Intake Form, Consent to Treatment, HIPAA Privacy Form, Patient Rights Form, Cancellation Policy, Notice to Payment)

☐ Obtain Medicare or other government-funded application and approval PTAN number for practice and each therapist (855I); Reassignment of individual therapists PTAN to practice (855R); Change in ownership/management (855I); Deactivation of PTANs (855R)

☐ DMERC contract and numbers (PTAN, NPI)

☐ EFT contract and procedures updated

☐ NPI numbers for practice, each therapist, and DME

☐ Contracts with third party payers current and on file

☐ Labor law review; overtime log, time alteration log, patient sign in log, time off log, holiday and benefit log, PTO log

☐ Current policy and documentation for part-time or full-time benefits

☐ Policy and Procedure Manual

☐ OSHA and universal safety policy and manual, and postings

☐ Chart review

☐ Outcome measurements

☐ Patient satisfaction surveys

☐ Equipment calibration service log

☐ Equipment and modalities maintenance log

☐ Emergency procedures

☐ Medical record and safety tracking procedures

☐ Employee contracts

☐ Billing
  o Prescription or referral, if indicated
  o Superbill
  o Supply sheets/costs
  o Evaluation/assessment documentation

(continued)

- o Daily encounter note (Time in/time out)
- o 30-day progress note
- o Discharge summary
- o Denial, restriction, and delay procedures
- o Scope of practice/Evidence-based support materials
- o Code restrictions noted
- o EOB posting procedures
- o Aging accounts procedures
- o Billing and coding changes retrieval procedures
- o Recertification/re-credentialing of therapists with payers

❏ Accounting
- o Income/expense daily, monthly
- o Budget
- o Payroll (see above reports required)
- o Independent contractors or per diem accounting
- o Shareholder accounting

❏ Human Resources
- o Hiring/firing procedures
- o Peer review
- o Wage increase
- o Benefits qualification
- o Employee handbook
- o Disciplinary actions/procedures
- o Staffing development/Staff meetings

❏ Marketing
- o Marketing strategies (business cards, brochures, ads, website, etc)
- o Marketing budget
- o Marketing tasks procedures (who, when, how often)

- Billing and coding: There are three general types of billing forms—HCFA-1500, the Uniform Bill, and the superbill. The first two types are mainly utilized for the federal insurance and grant funds such as Medicare and Medicaid. However, they can also be used in private practice for other payment systems.

  The superbill is a billing form that indicates which types of services were provided, their billing codes and price, and product information. The client generally pays for services and products at the time they were received, and personally submits the superbill to his or her payer system for reimbursement. Services and products are represented by codes for all of the billing types mentioned. The diagnosis codes describe the client's medical condition or disease. ICD-9-CM is the diagnostic coding system generally used. Procedure codes describe specific services such as an evaluation or therapeutic exercise. Examples of procedures coding systems include CPT and HCPCS. The coding systems are usually updated annually by the American Medical Association. Keep in mind that billing and coding must also meet HIPAA compliance.

- *Provider network:* This is an organization formed to acquire managed care contracts for its members (ie, private practitioners such as occupational and physical therapists). It markets to vendors (third-party payers) for health care service contracts. The network may be organized either by a payer such as an insurance company, or by private organizations such as Preferred Therapy Providers of America (PTPN). In general terms, its goal is to negotiate for you to third-party payers instead of you personally contracting with them yourself. Third-party payers are interested in keeping health care costs down. Therefore, they often prefer to work through provider networks who offer competitive reimbursement pricing.[4]

Workflow Management Checklist

Administrative management
- ❏ Hours of operation
- ❏ Scheduling
- ❏ Employee functions
- ❏ Marketing

Information management
- ❏ Customer service
- ❏ Patient intake
- ❏ Communication with referral sources and payers
- ❏ Other front office tasks

Regulatory compliance
- ❏ Policies and procedures
- ❏ Health care rules and regulations

Documentation compliance
- ❏ Referral/prescription
- ❏ Medical records
- ❏ Client care/interventions
- ❏ Treatment protocols

Personnel
- ❏ Supervision
- ❏ Professional development and training

Financial management
- ❏ Bookkeeping and accounting
- ❏ Coding and billing

Legal compliance
- ❏ Agreements
- ❏ Government filings
- ❏ Employment policies
- ❏ Corporate records

You have to apply and pay service fees to the provider network if you choose to belong. If you are planning on performing coding and billing on your own, it is very important that you learn the appropriate billing codes. If you billed inappropriately, whether you knew it or not, you could be charged with fraud. There are classes, courses, and books available to help educate you on health care billing. Talk to colleagues to determine what they are doing for billing. Many practices outsource their billing to an individual medical biller or medical billing services.

Facility Management Checklist

- ☐ Signage
- ☐ Lighting
- ☐ Interior walls
- ☐ Emergency systems
- ☐ Evacuation plans
- ☐ Storage of materials
- ☐ Equipment maintenance
- ☐ Electronics/electrical
- ☐ Computer networking/upgrades
- ☐ Phone systems
- ☐ Security systems
- ☐ Supply inventory/upgrade
- ☐ Furniture and décor condition
- ☐ ADA compliance
- ☐ Parking spaces/handicap
- ☐ Overall safety

High Risk Areas:

_____

_____

Needs Repairs:

_____

_____

To Schedule:

_____

_____

To Do:

_____

_____

Tips and Tools

Corporate compliance or health care compliance is a "good faith" plan to meet health care standards, regulations, and guidelines established by various organizational bodies such as the governmental agencies, AOTA, APTA, or state associations, state licensure, and similar regulatory bodies within your practice. Compliance programs are created for the main purpose of preventing fraud and abuse by implementing the seven steps provided by the Office of Inspector General (OIG).

The seven components of a compliance program are:

1. Establish written policies and procedures, including code of conduct.
2. Designate a compliance officer and contact person.
3. Conduct training and education on practice ethics, policies and procedures, and applicable laws and regulations.
4. Conduct internal monitoring, auditing, and reporting to detect non-compliance and specific risk areas.
5. Develop open lines of communication with staff and patients to allow expression of issues and misconduct.
6. Develop and enforce disciplinary standards.
7. Respond to identified problems and take appropriate course of action.

Learn more at www.complianceinfo.com or www.hcca-info.org.

STEP 3: BUILD YOUR MANAGEMENT SKILLS AND STANDARDS OF CARE

As we learned in Chapter 1, entrepreneurs, managers, and leaders share several of the same characteristics. Now these characteristics need to become building blocks for building management skills. Here are the characteristics that you will need to develop:

- Make a commitment to change and learning.
- Develop an ability to embrace error.
- Be willing to encourage dissent and engage in creative resolution.
- Engage in "reflective backtalk" or critique.
- Be open to others with different or better ideas.
- Act with a clear and accountable plan for change.
- Constantly improve the ability to generate and sustain trust.

As a new manager or owner, you will need to develop your overall approach to both your practice and your staff. There are several theories on what the best type of "leadership" approach is. You may want to invest some time and money on reading and learning more about building your leadership skills. Furthermore, how you lead is often a reflection of your previous work and relationship experiences. We recommend you take a look at your DATA worksheet from Chapter 1 and get reacquainted with who you are first. Examine how you manage other areas of your life. Which of the many operational tasks are you going to perform personally, and which will you outsource? Make a copy of the "Management and Operations Checklist" and begin to circle the items you have the skills and interest to perform yourself, then highlight the tasks that you will hire someone else to do. Begin to establish your organizational chart that we discussed in Chapter 2. Hiring therapy staff and other types of personnel will require you to become familiar with the labor laws within your state. There are several other tasks on the management and operations checklist that will require that you confer with an expert in small business laws. Make sure to ask about required work benefits, overtime, wage guidelines, and hiring and firing standards. Also, contact your state association and network with your peers about performance reviews, salary rates, and other important benchmarks dependent on local standards of practice rather than national benchmarks. Contact your state licensure board or certification board to read and understand your scope of practice, supervisory guidelines, and other practice regulations. Keep in mind your payer, network provider, or other certification agencies will also have their own required operational guidelines you will have to comply with.

The general rule of thumb in management is to follow "standards of practice." This refers to both regulated and "usual, customary, and reasonable" practice operations that are given in this text. You are expected to implement the basic foundational operational tasks that comply with regulations and are typical of all therapists with your same level of education and skills. However, the concept of managing within our therapy framework and within our standards of practice is now evolving into the term "evidence-based practice." Evidence-based practice (EBP) is the use of systematic research review to formally gather and synthesize information from research findings to determine best practice standards.[6] Managers use evidence for decision making and to develop and support effective clinical programs, efficient assessments, and interventions. For example, ask yourself: "Are my therapy interventions supported by research or outcomes that lead to providing services that are most proven or recognized to be most effective for that particular diagnosis, or some set of patient parameters?" You can also think of them as treatment protocols or practice guidelines.

There are five steps in an EBP[6]:

1. Ask the question.
2. Search and sort the research. Analyze existing literature and articles from various databases.
3. Critically appraise the evidence. Discern the level of research, appraise content, apply critical reasoning, and decide on "best practice" interventions.
4. Apply to practice and either accept or reject. Implement and perform the intervention based on the findings, and become competent in intervention.
5. Conduct a self assessment. Apply outcome measurements such as pre- and post-assessments.

The benefits of integrating the framework of evidence-based practice into your business operations is to increase revenues through better insurance coverage and better customer satisfaction. Improve your quality of care with performing higher standards of service interventions. Improve your service efficiency by reaching the short- and long-term treatment goals sooner and better.

To implement the five steps of EBP within your practice, you will need to consider these important elements: Is your practice or organization logistically and strategically equipped to support the best standard? Which method of implementation results in quality of care? Is the staff competent, and is it worth your time and efforts of the overall organization? For example, studies show that peer support and exercise is more effective than just exercise alone for increasing community integration in stroke survivors. However, your practice space is not large enough to implement group support sessions, and group sessions would require additional staffing or supervising. Therefore, you decide to rent additional space at the local YMCA once a week to hold group support sessions and ask caregivers to attend to assist you. You, the manager, will need to apply the five steps and use critical reasoning on what is best for your clients, your staff, and your operations.

This process also applies to the choices you make in regard to your systems documentation and implementation. The manager and operations checklist is your "standards" or operational guideline to begin implementing standards of management. Thus, evidence-based management begins by applying the five steps of EBP to your operations. Besides the operational checklist, you will need to develop methods and skills in socializing your company's values and vision, and in promoting communication and collaboration within your practice as well as out in the community that you serve. If you work for yourself, you will need the same managerial and leadership skills to sustain your practice and professional livelihood. Seek out additional information and build your management skills in EBP and evidence-based management through the resources at your national associations and other resources found at the end of this chapter.

Tips and Tools

The implementation of a quality assurance program is often required of provider networks and some credentialing agencies. It is basically a systematic way to identify potential problem areas or risks inherent in practice operations that need to be regularly examined and resolved in order to assure high standards of care.

The objectives of a quality assurance problem are:

- To identify and appraise all of the practice's activities concerned with client care
- To promote and assist in the development of competency-based standards of performance for all staff positions, and to assist in evaluation performance based on these standards
- To identify and address areas of substandard care or problems that could interfere with the provision of quality care, and to discuss these areas with appropriate staff
- To assess problems objectively for causes, effects, extent, and previous remedial action, and to set priorities for investigation and resolution
- To recommend corrective action
- To monitor any problems to resolution

These objectives are implemented and resourced by several operational tasks:

- Peer reviews
- Monthly chart reviews
- Annual performance evaluations
- Client complaints and unusual occurrence reports
- Client satisfaction surveys
- Miscellaneous other documents such as staff meeting minutes, fiscal reports, review of policies and procedures, staffing reports, and any audits

Step 4: Promote Professional Competency and Code of Ethics

Two important aspects of building a solid management foundation are promoting professional competency and ethical behavior. You will continuously be asked to demonstrate competency throughout the operations of your business and professional life. You will also expect that of your employees. Start with asking three questions:

1. What does it mean to be competent?
2. Who determines whether someone is competent?
3. Who is responsible for ensuring whether someone is competent?

Competency is an individual's performance in a particular situation that implies that the person is capable of performing a behavior or task as measured against a specific criterion.[7] Professional development is one way of developing new skills, more roles, and responsibilities. The national and state associations have valuable resources for achieving professional development.

Determining whether someone is competent can fall under several entities. You, as the owner and manager, may determine that your employees need to have a certain skill set in order to meet the qualifications of the positions they hold. The licensure and regulations board determines competency requirements for entry-level professional, board certifications, and so forth. Other accreditation bodies such as NBCOT or provider networks may require demonstration of your competency through your professional development units or continued educational units requirements. The same group of entities is also responsible for ensuring competency. Overall, the standards of continuing competency involve having knowledge and demonstrating critical reasoning, interpersonal skills, performance skills, and ethical reasoning.

Competency and professional development are important for several reasons:

- To avoid consequences of ineffective assessments, interventions, or improper service delivery
- To avoid loss of license or certification
- To avoid and prevent lawsuits

The success and sustainability of your business is dependent on demonstrating competency. Make sure that you and your staff are taking the time and the money to upgrade your skills to accommodate the demands of EBP, standards of care, and appropriate delivery of services.

Managers need to be prepared to face all of the ethical challenges that will come with operating your own business within our present health care environment. Performing the first two steps of this chapter will assist in implementing the documentation and tools to support clinical and operational efficacy. However, every decision you make about your practice and within your organization represents an ethical statement or belief. There are three major ethical functions of a manager[7]:

1. Keep faith with the tenets, principles, and standards of the profession.
2. Preserve the integrity of the professional community, obtain and maintain accreditations and licensure, and admit qualified students to the profession.
3. Ensure integrity of the individual practitioners and establish a culture of introspection and self review.

The state and national associations have published ethical guidelines, which you should purchase or print out for your learning and implementation. Keep in mind that we may know what we can or cannot do or perform according to our scope of practice, our selection of services, or our supervisory guidelines, but many of the agencies and even our clients that we will come in contact with won't. Don't neglect to live up to these standards of care despite the complexity of operating your own business.

Tips and Tools

Business operational success can be divided into four areas[8]:

1. Recruitment and Scheduling of Patients

    "For marketing and scheduling systems to be successful, they should be: centralized, consistent, accessible, understandable, have staff level control and staff level planning, and they should capture information that is used in subsequent business processes such as documentation and billing."

2. Treatment Intervention and Documentation of Care

    "For treatment intervention and documentation systems to be successful, they should be: data-based, evidence-driven, real time decision making, reflective of complex decision making, reflective of professional level skills, accessible, based on each episode of interaction, and they should provide readily available reports."

3. Billing and Management of Finances

    Billing and accounting need to be performed regularly, monitored for accuracy and compliance, audited periodically for changes and updates, and adjusted as needed to policy and contract changes.

4. Analysis of Outcomes

    Outcomes should measure both business and clinical operations and services, reassess and redirect according to analysis of data, compare to rehab community benchmarks, and work toward evidence-based medicine interventions and practice standards.

CHAPTER 5 SUMMARY

Implementation of your health care practice and business plan involves multiple activities that happen all year round and indefinitely. It is important to find the strategies, tools, and network of peers and experts to assist you.

Step 1: Gather Advice and Consultation from Experts

_____

_____

_____

Step 2: Complete Your Operational Infrastructure
   ❏ Perform the start-up tasks checklist.
   ❏ Obtain and implement your clinical documentation.
   ❏ Obtain and implement your systems documentation.
   ❏ Perform the management and operations checklist.
   ❏ Perform the workflow management checklist.
   ❏ Perform the facility management checklist.
   ❏ Review the various operations and management template tools in Appendix D.

Step 3: Build Your Management Skills and Standards of Care
   ❏ Continue to gain knowledge and implement evidence-based practice.

Step 4: Promote Professional Competency and Code of Ethics
   ❏ Continue to gain knowledge and implement professional competency and code of ethics.
   ❏ Seek out additional resources on management and leadership models.
   ❏ Seek out peers and experts for support and advice.

Action Plan
   ❏ Perform the documentation self-assessment in Appendix E.
   ❏ Perform the productivity assessment in Appendix F.

References

1. Acquaviva J. Documentation of occupational therapy services. *The Occupational Therapy Manager.* 4th ed. AOTA Press; 2003:375-384.

2. Goldstein V. *Employment Law.* Deerfield Beach, FL: Made E-Z Products, Inc; 2000.

3. Acquaviva J. *Effective Documentation for Occupational Therapy.* 2nd ed. Bethesda, MD: American Occupational Therapy Association, Inc; 1998.

4. Glassman S. Purchasing power in numbers. *Advance for Physical Therapists and PT Assistants* [serial online]. 1997. Available at: http://physical-therapy.advanceweb.com/Editorial/Search/AViewer.aspx?AN=PT_p10.html&AD=11-17-1997. Accessed October 30, 2008.

5. Young H. Taking stock: analyzing your business relationships and billing practices can help you avoid potential fraud risks. *Advance for Physical Therapists and PT Assistants* [serial online]. 13(12):11. Available at: http://physical-therapy.advanceweb.com/Editorial/Search/AViewer.aspx?AN=PT_02jun10_ptp11.html&AD=06-10-2002. Accessed October 30, 2008.

6. Abreu B. Evidence-based practice. *The Occupational Therapy Manager.* 4th ed. AOTA Press; 2003:351-374.

7. Moyers P, Hinojosa J. Continuing competency. *The Occupational Therapy Manager.* 4th ed. AOTA Press; 2003:463-489.

8. Kovacek P. The four horsemen of rehab success. *Advance for Physical Therapists and PT Assistants* [serial online]. 2000;11(16):5. Available at: http://physical-therapy.advanceweb.com/Editorial/Search/AViewer.aspx?AN=PT_p5.html&AD=08-07-2000. Accessed October 30, 2008.

Suggested Reading

American Occupational Therapy Association. Entrepreneurial resource columns. Available at: http://www.aota.org/Pubs/OTP/1997-2007/Columns/ER.aspx. Accessed December 30, 2008.

American Occupational Therapy Association Press. *The Occupational Therapy Manager.* 4th ed. Bethesda, MD: American Occupational Therapy Association, Inc; 2003

American Physical Therapy Association. *Law & Liability. Part 1: Liability Issues.* Alexandria, VA: American Physical Therapy Association; 1999.

American Physical Therapy Association. *Law & Liability. Part 2: Professional Issues.* Alexandria, VA: American Physical Therapy Association; 1999.

Bassett J. Finding the perfect fit: hiring the right clinicians and office staff can mean success and failure. *Advance for Physical Therapists and PT Assistants.* 2002;13(16):8.

Coleman D. *Business: The Ultimate Resource.* Cambridge, MA: Perseus Book Groups; 2002.

Cook C, Cook A. Meet the challenge: by staying billing savvy, you can avoid Medicare denials. *Advance for Directors in Rehabilitation* [serial online]. 2003;12(5):19. Available at: http://rehabilitation-director.advanceweb.com/Editorial/Search/AViewer.aspx?AN=DR_03may1_drp19.html&AD=05-01-2003. Accessed October 30, 2008.

Curtis K. *The Physical Therapist's Guide to Health Care.* Thorofare, NJ: SLACK Incorporated; 1999.

Diffendal J. Dressing your clinic for success. *Advance for Occupational Therapy Practitioners.* 2002;18(5):15-16.

Fazio L. *Developing Occupation-Centered Program for the Community: A Workbook for Students and Professionals.* 2nd ed. Upper Saddle River, NJ: Prentice Hall; 2007.

Fleischmann K. Should you outsource billing operations, or keep them in-house? *Advance for Physical Therapists and PT Assistants.* 2007;19(10):34.

Frohriep E. Risky business: therapists should complete an incident report after every adverse patient event. *Advance for Directors in Rehabilitation.* 2007;16(5):15.

Glennon T. Putting on your business hat. *OT Practice.* 2007;Feb(3):23-25.

Hack L, Hillyer R, Kovacek P. *Business Skills In Physical Therapy: Defining Your Business.* Alexandria, VA: American Physical Therapy Association; 2003.

Hardeman L. The heart of an entrepreneur. *OT Practice.* 2007;Jan(1):13-15.

Jacobs K, Logigian M. *Functions of a Manager in Occupational Therapy.* 3rd ed. Thorofare, NJ: SLACK Incorporated; 1999.

Jusinski L. Career center: connecting with generation Y. *Advance for Occupational Therapy Practitioners* [serial online]. 2007. Available at: http://occupational-therapy.advanceweb.com/Editorial/Search/AViewer.aspx?CC=103767. Accessed October 30, 2008.

LaGrossa J. Teaching evidence based practice. *Advance for Occupational Therapy Practitioners.* 2006;22(18):17.

Law M. *Evidence-Based Rehabilitation: A Guide to Practice.* Thorofare, NJ: SLACK Incorporated; 2002.

Lewis DK, Kovacek P. *Business Skills in Physical Therapy: Legal Issues*. Alexandria, VA: American Physical Therapy Association; 2002.

Martin P. On the mark: financial and operating growth strategies can solidify your practice. *Advance for Directors in Rehabilitation*. 2002;11(8):13-14. Available at: http://rehabilitation-director.advanceweb.com/Editorial/Search/AViewer.aspx?AN=DR_02aug1_drp13.html&AD=08-01-2002. Accessed October 30, 2008.

Moyers P. Errors in occupational therapy. *OT Practice*. 2005;8:18.

Piersol C, Ehrlick P. *Home Health Practice: A Guide for the Occupational Therapist*. Bisbee, AZ: Imaginart International, Inc; 2000.

Pozgar G. *Legal Aspects of Health Care Administration*. 10th ed. Sudbury, MA: Jones and Bartlett Publishers; 2006.

Rooks F. Negligence includes more than improper patient care: is your practice protected? *Advance for Directors in Rehabilitation*. 2007;17(4):11.

Scott R. *Legal Aspects of Documenting Patient Care*. 3rd ed. Sudbury, MA: Jones and Bartlett Publishers, Inc; 2006.

Slater D. The ethics of productivity. *OT Practice*. 2006;Oct:17-20.

Sohnen-Moe CM. *Business Mastery: A Guide for Creating a Fulfilling, Thriving Business and Keeping it Successful*. 4th ed. Tucson, AZ: Sohnen-Moe Associates, Inc; 2007.

RELATED RESOURCES

American Occupational Therapy Association
Fax-On-Request for information on multiple practice topics including continuing education, education, practice ethics, products and publications, reimbursement and regulatory policies.
(800) 701-7735

American Physical Therapy Association
Fax-On-Demand for information on several practice topics such as continuing education, education, government affairs, insurance plans, reimbursement, specialist certifications, and research demographics.
(800) 399-2782

MEDICARE RESOURCES

American Occupational Therapy Association. *Skilled Therapy: Medicare Coverage Guidelines for the Continuum of Care*. Vol 1 and 2. Bethesda, MD: American Occupational Therapy Association, Inc.

FINANCIAL MANAGEMENT 6

John Richmond, CLU, ChFC

Tammy Richmond, MS, OTRL

CHAPTER OBJECTIVES

✓ Understand accounting basics.
✓ Manage your cash flow.
✓ Improve your profitability and manage your risks.
✓ Understand the basics to billing and reimbursement.

[NOTE: The information presented in this chapter should not be interpreted as specific accounting and financial advice for any particular health care provider. Personal financial advice should be performed by a personal accountant, financial advisor, or tax attorney, and it should be based on applicable state and federal laws.]

Financial management of any business is the lifeblood of the organization. In other words, financial management of an organization has to be understood and managed—not in detail, but conceptually at all times. It is important to keep good recordkeeping practices and to hire a professional bookkeeper, accountant, or tax service.

Hiring professional assistance for monthly record reconciliations, filing appropriate tax forms on a timely basis, and then providing you with all of those reports in a clear, concise way each month of the year and in the year end statement is worth the business expense and the tax write-off for that expense. You need your energy and attitude to run, enhance, and grow your business. By creating this team mentality, you can also rely on their input when considering new business decisions. The bookkeeping service will keep you out of tax trouble as well as provide you with the most current accurate tax information. Ignorance is not acceptable to the IRS. To make matters worse, the penalties levied for mistakes are often worse than the actual tax amount due, and that may leave you at risk for additional scrutiny.

There are four steps to good financial management:

Step 1: Understand accounting basics.
Step 2: Manage your cash flow.
Step 3: Improve your profitability and manage your risks.
Step 4: Understand the basics to billing and reimbursement.

STEP 1: UNDERSTAND ACCOUNTING BASICS

Understanding accounting basics starts with defining some basic terms:

- *Accounts payable:* The debts that your business owes, such as your bills and credit card balances.
- *Accounts receivable:* The amounts you are owed by your clients, insurance carriers, or others for services and products.
- *Cash basis:* A method of accounting in which income is recorded when the cash is actually received, not when you bill it or invoice it. Expenses are recorded when actually paid, not when the invoice is received or the services are rendered. This method is less complicated than the accrual basis of accounting.
- *Accrual basis:* The method of accounting in which you record income and expenses at the time they are incurred, not when you actually receive the income for the expense.
- *Cash flow:* Actual income and expenses moving in and out of a business.

✛ *Establish a Bookkeeping System*

In Chapter 3, you learned how to create and estimate your start-up costs, operating costs budget, income statements, and other financial documents. Now that your rehab business is up and running, you will have to manage the daily expenses and income items. This is best handled by performing regular bookkeeping activities.

The objectives of bookkeeping include[1]:

- Allow monitoring of your business progress.
- Assist in preparing the financial statements.
- Assist in identifying the source of receipts.
- Allow tracking of deductible expenses.
- Assist in preparing tax returns.
- Support items reported on your tax returns.

Overall, your bookkeeping system needs to record and report gross income, deductions, and credits. There are four main categories of business accounting support documents[1]:

1. *Gross receipts:* Those income receipts that you receive from your business such as payments on your invoices, cash and credit card receipts, bank deposit slips, and check stubs.

2. *Purchases:* Documents that demonstrate the amount of a business purchase such as cancelled checks, credit card summaries, or receipts.

3. *Expenses:* Documents that show the costs to operate your business such as receipts, account statements, and invoices.

4. *Assets:* Documentation of property leased or purchased for your business to verify annual depreciation, costs, or sales expenses.

Conceivably, all of your bookkeeping needs can be met with a computer accounting software package such as QuickBooks by Intuit. Typical accounting software contains four main activity areas:

1. Sales and customers
2. Purchases and vendors
3. Checking and credit cards
4. Taxes and accountant

Financial forms such as the profit/loss statement, balance sheet, cash flow statement, etc, are automatically generated for you as you enter your business financial data. Most software programs also allow you to generate business checks, tax forms, and many other business-related financial documents. Taking a class to learn how to implement and use your accounting software program is highly recommended. If you have hired or plan on hiring an accountant to assist you, ask which software brand he or she prefers. Since you will need to share files and figures, most accountants prefer their clients to utilize the same accounting software.

If, for whatever reason, you decide not to purchase accounting software, then purchase a general ledger or business journal that will allow you to keep track of your income and business expenses. Some business ledgers found in business supply stores already contain itemized pages of business expense categories or specific business expense items. The items that you listed in your cash flow statement within your business plan can act as a guide to income and expense line items. Establish a general financial bookkeeping schedule to assist in effective financial management.

Example of Financial Bookkeeping Schedule

Daily Activities
- ❏ Collect payments from clients for services rendered.
- ❏ Perform client invoicing for services/products.
- ❏ Check inventory.
- ❏ Complete daily charge slips for rehab services/products or supplies provided.
- ❏ If self-billing or in-house billing, complete billing form and send.

Weekly Activities
- ❏ Deposit accounts receivables, including third-party payments and copayments.
- ❏ Enter any purchases made.
- ❏ If outsourcing billing, send explanation of benefits (EOB), charge slips, and other related billing info to the medical biller.

Bimonthly Activities
- ❏ Send out payroll and post expenses.
- ❏ Pay bills and post expenses.
- ❏ Post EOBs, check over denials, and statements from payers.
- ❏ Resubmit claims and invoice clients.

Monthly Activities
- ❏ Balance business checking and savings account.
- ❏ Pay loans and leases.
- ❏ Total and balance accounts receivable and accounts payable.
- ❏ Check client accounts for balance due and send out statements.
- ❏ Complete medical billing AR (accounts receivable) report, balances, denials.
- ❏ Have a consultation with the accountant and financial advisor.

Quarterly Activities
- ❏ Pay estimated taxes.
- ❏ Pay sales and use tax.
- ❏ Update cash flow projections.
- ❏ Audit coding changes, billing procedures.
- ❏ Have a consultation with the accountant and financial advisor.

Yearly Activities
- ❏ Pay all invoices and other expenses for current year deductions.
- ❏ Prepare end-of-year financial statements and balance and income statements.
- ❏ Organize supportive documents for the accountant.
- ❏ Meet with the financial advisor for end-of-year investments, tax strategies, and establishing funds.
- ❏ Complete medical billing end-of-year AR report.

✛ *Open Up a Business Checking Account and a Business Credit Card*

The two-checkbook system! The two-checkbook system provides two main benefits:
1.   Accurate recordkeeping
2.   Separation of money between business expenses and personal expenses

The two-checkbook system requires that you set up a checking account in the name of your business entity and continue to use your personal checking account for personal expenses only. All income generated from the business in any shape or form is to be deposited into this business account. Since the checkbook acts as your most basic source of recordkeeping information, be sure to record the type of expense, the source of any revenues, and the types of expenses for checks drawn on the account. Checks for personal use should be recorded first as business payroll, and then deposited into your personal account.

Only checks that are for legitimate business expenses should be written out of the business checkbook. Avoid writing out checks to cash. As a general rule, all business revenue should be deposited as soon as conveniently possible.

Reconcile your business checking account when you receive your monthly bank statements to determine any errors or omissions and any incorrect financial balances.

Obtain a business credit card instead of utilizing an existing personal credit card. The advantages include easier purchase tracking for record keeping, credit limits that allow for bigger purchases with monthly payments, online purchases, and value-added services.

✛ *Manage Your Business Receipts*

One of the easier but often mishandled financial tasks to perform is developing a way to manage your business income and expense receipts.

Income Receipts

The most common type of income in a rehab business is accounts receivable for health care services and related retail products. This includes copayments, third-party and other payer payments, and cash or credit card payments for your rehab business services and products. If you are selling retail products, you will generally have to apply for a state resale license to charge and collect sales tax on the retail product sales, and remit these taxes on a monthly, quarterly, or annual basis. Posting all income as it comes in daily on your bookkeeping software or general ledger is vital to keeping accurate records and avoiding miscalculating your operating budget and rehab business cash flow.

Expense Receipts

Yes, you should save any and all purchase receipts, credit card expense statements, expense invoices, bank statements, savings accounts statements, and any other type of document that indicates your rehab business spent money on an item.

Federal tax deductions are business-related expenses that can be legally deducted from your business gross income. They are often referred to as "ordinary and necessary."[2] The United States Congress enacts tax laws into the tax code, which the IRS interprets and then codifies, that identify which expenses will be allowed as a deduction against gross income. Common examples of business deductions include:
*   State, local, and property taxes
*   Medical expenses and health insurance
*   Casualty and loss expenses
*   Business travel and educational costs
*   Purchases financed by business loans or credit cards
*   Professional membership fees
*   Utilities
*   Rent
*   Charitable contributions

The type and amount of business deduction allowances vary accordingly to many different tax law parameters. Tax deductions of home-based rehab businesses need to be especially understood and carefully handled because there are several conditions to be met. Get professional assistance and advice.

If you have accounting software, enter the business expense receipt amount under the specified expense category, and keep all of your receipts divided into monthly folders or a similar type of organizer. You may need to be able to support the expenses claimed on your tax return by presenting the original source documents in the event of a tax audit.

✛ *Organize Your Financial Statements*

All financial documents need to be kept and organized to allow easy retrieval, verification, and analysis of your rehab business' financial picture. You learned about several types of financial documents in Chapter 3. Depending on your business plan objectives, you may have created an operating cost statement and a cash flow statement.

Your operating costs statement (see Chapter 3) reports your main expense categories and variables that reflect your accounts payable. These variables should be customized to your specific rehab business expenses. The monthly costs of your expenses are posted into your cash flow projection statement (see Chapter 3). The ending cash balance represents your beginning cash balance plus deposits, less your expenses paid out. This amount will be the following month's beginning balance.

Your operating budget requires that you enter amounts from your supportive documents. General supportive financial documents to keep include:

- Inventory lists
- Bank statements and cancelled checks
- Fixed assets logs (items that are depreciated)
- Accounts payables and accounts receivables
- Client accounts and invoices
- Loan statements and documents
- Any other financial statement, investments, etc
- Tax returns
- Tax filings
- Tax records, payroll, etc
- Any other tax documents

Financial documents must be retained for 3 to 7 years to comply with IRS tax policies. There are some records that should be kept permanently such as your payroll records and depreciation schedules. Check with your accountant or tax advisor, or visit www.irs.gov.

Special Considerations for the Rehab Professional

A common mistake made by health care providers going into their own rehab business is not spending enough time researching and creating their financial documents with accurate numbers. Go back to your start-up costs, operating costs, and pricing of your services and products, and ask yourself these questions:

- What purchases do I absolutely need to make now, and which can be purchased on an as-needed basis?

  _____

- How many hours do I (or employees) need to work, or how much do I need to charge to cover my expenses?

  _____

- Should I lease or purchase some of my bigger expenses?

  _____

Talk to existing rehab business owners, accountants, and area colleagues to assist you in answering these questions easily and accurately.

Tips and Tools

Hiring a tax accountant or certified public accountant (CPA) is vital to the success of any small business. Tax laws and regulations change often and require professional interpretation. The important considerations when hiring an accountant to assist you include:

- Works with small businesses
- Is licensed or certified
- Has business insurance and references
- Has good communication skills
- Is available for continuous support and services
- Fees represent services
- Has an excellent understanding of tax laws, regulations, and resources to tax changes

There are other similar professionals such as bookkeepers, tax lawyers, and tax return preparers that differ by qualifications, services, skills, and experiences. You will need to find someone who is best qualified to meet your accounting and tax needs. Again, the best way to find an accountant is generally through personal referrals. Fees for services may also differ from hourly fees to flat fees. Having a written agreement or at least an agreeable fee schedule will avoid misinformation and potential financial disputes.

STEP 2: MANAGE YOUR CASH FLOW

Here are a couple of professional financial truisms:

- The first purpose of a business is not to be profitable. The first purpose of a business is to provide a benefit or service to a consumer that he or she cannot provide for him- or herself as well as you can, in which the consumer is able to recognize this benefit as valuable and pay for it.
- Second, it is not as important for a business, especially a new business, to be profitable as it is for it to have cash flow. Cash flow requires customers right from the start, and that is where you want to spend your time and energy.

Managing your cash flow depends on understanding three financial terms:

1. Purchase or acquisition expenses
2. Fixed expenses
3. Variable expenses

Purchase expenses are those business items that you paid for and own, and that you will deduct or depreciate over time according to the amortization schedule provided by the IRS. These become your assets. Examples of purchase expenses include:

- Initial inventory of supplies
- Office equipment (in your home or office)
- Therapy equipment
- Lab coats for you or an employee
- Business vehicle

Fixed expenses, also called "overhead expenses," are costs that do not vary from month to month based on usage and are the most critical expense area to watch. This is the area where a bad mistake seriously affects the viability of the business. Fixed expenses are normally accompanied by contracts and monthly payments obligating you to pay, and there are usually negative consequences if you don't pay on time. Examples of fixed expenses include:

- Leased equipment
- Rental space
- Services
- Hired employees
- Business loans

Fixed expenses are necessary, so be very careful when you enter into those obligations. Hire a lawyer to read through any contracts and explain your financial obligations and risk exposure. You can get into some terrible expenditure situations if you don't understand contract laws. You must remember that your signature obligates you, your assets, and the assets of your estate to pay.

The third kind of expense is variable expenses, and these are usually controllable and fluctuate with volume of services and products being utilized. They have a direct relationship with cash flow because they represent potential rehab business profitability. Examples would include:

- Telephone usage (not the equipment or lines because those are fixed)
- Postage
- Advertising
- Direct mail
- Fuel for an automobile (if it is utilized for work)
- Therapy and office supplies
- Salaries and benefits
- Marketing

Variable expenses will increase or decrease depending on the activity in your business. Variable expenses can be thought of as variable investments. If you try something to improve your business and it does not work, you can stop and try something else. The consequence isn't anything that will be detrimental to the life of your business. No harm done! Always keep track of what you are doing and its effectiveness. With variable expenses, they are usually 100% tax-deductible during the calendar year you are incurring the expense, so think of the IRS helping you out a little by allowing the tax deduction. Be reminded, however, that the IRS will help themselves back when you become profitable.

It is important to divide the business expense items into the three expense categories because you want to be able to understand how profit is made and where costs can be controlled. Most are fully tax-deductible for your business. A word of advice here is to allow your business to provide you, the business owner, with quality items needed to conduct your business while deducting these expenses against the business revenues. As your business grows and has a better cash flow or profitability, continued reinvestment will provide the financial security for a successful business and enhance your growth potential.

Special Considerations for the Rehab Professional

Increasing your profitability and managing risks require that you learn how to maximize your health care accounts receivables. Here are 14 suggestions to achieve maximum cash flow[3]:

1. Make sure you collect all necessary client information in detail before the initial evaluation.
2. Use proper CPT and ICD-9 codes.
3. Collect copayments and the coinsurance amount at each visit.
4. Keep your clients informed from the start about their financial responsibility.
5. Make sure clients with personal injury cases from auto injuries have an adequate money limit.
6. Make sure to find out before beginning treatment if there is pending litigation.
7. Know the laws and policies regarding claim denials and reviews.
8. Make sure you have an organized financial tracking system.
9. Review all explanations of payments to make sure proper reimbursement is made.
10. Review current managed care contracts to determine whether they still benefit the business.
11. Keep the staff and clients informed of any reimbursement changes.
12. Compare current billing to electronic billing to make a better decision about in-house versus outsourcing billing tasks.
13. Know your recourse for legitimate unresolved money balances.
14. Be persistent.

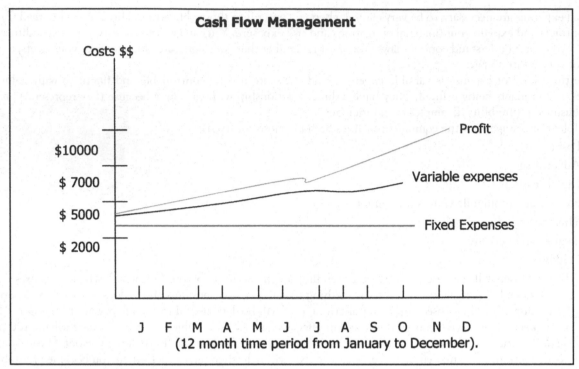

Figure 6-1. Profitable cash flow management.

STEP 3: IMPROVE YOUR PROFITABILITY AND MANAGE YOUR RISKS

Your ultimate rehab business financial goal is to be successful and make a profit. A typical successful business financial graph will show fixed and variable expenses at their starting cost level point in numbers of dollars. Your rehab business financial management objective is to make the cash flow (income) meet the fixed and variable expenses, and to eventually exceed those amounts to show a profit (Figure 6-1). To make a profit, you will need to learn how to improve your profitability through improving your cash flow avenues and managing your risks.

✛ Improve Your Cash Flow

There are several avenues to improving your cash flow. Closely monitoring all of your financial parameters is crucial to running a successful rehab business.

Improving your cash flow involves several objectives:
- Monitoring accounts receivables and accounts payables
- Investing in expenses (tax deductions)
- Building and maintaining a cash reserve
- Investing surplus cash into profitable returns
- Reinvesting back into your rehab business

Monitor Accounts Receivables and Accounts Payables

One of the first and foremost fundamental items in improving your cash flow is from conducting careful recordkeeping of all revenues and expenses. Avoid falling behind in identifying, recording, and tracking incoming money from all of your various sources and outgoing expenses.

Invest in Expenses (Tax Deductions)

Look for positive ways to invest in your rehab business that will cause increasing cash flow. These are generally your variable expenses (ie, those items that are tax-deductible).

Depending on your business organization type (eg, corporation versus sole proprietorship), you will realize that gross income is not what requires your attention, and net income does. You increase your net cash flow by legitimately buying rehab business items through the business financial funds and deducting those expenses from your gross revenue.

This lowers your tax bracket and, therefore, lowers your income taxes owed, yet it provides you with an avenue of being able to provide quality services and products. Laptop computers, printers, copiers, office supplies, therapy supplies, business vehicles, phones, furniture, and numerous other items that you need to operate and perform your rehab business services are good examples of legitimate business purchases that are tax-deductible.

Meet with an accountant and determine what types of business purchases qualify for tax deductions and the percentage of the write off. Avoid making business purchases that cannot benefit your rehab business and cannot be proven as necessary for rehab business operations such as deducting large restaurant and entertainment expense receipts. Also, remember that some of these items have a limited life according to the IRS depreciation tables, and you can then take them over personally for the salvage value that is recaptured on your business tax. Professional assistance is a must for understanding tax deductions and other write-offs with more complicated legal structures such as corporations and partnerships.

Build and Maintain a Cash Reserve

When building cash reserves, be aware of how your business organization is established. Your accountant and tax advisor can assist you with cash reserves. You should also understand the relationship and importance of cash flow as opposed to profitability in the early stages of business. The goal, depending on your type of business, is to build up between 3 to 6 months' reserves that equal your business' fixed and variable expenses according to your monthly financial statements to act as an emergency fund.

Invest Surplus Cash Into Profitable Returns

After you have met the 3 to 6 month cash reserve amount, address how you can make your money work for you. Keeping too much in a cash position (eg, in the checking account or in a money market with check writing privileges) is not putting your money to work for you.

There are several ways to accomplish this.

- Tax-exempt funds: investment funds that earn tax-exempt interest (ie, municipal bonds or mutual funds).
- Tax deferment funds: investment funds that allow income tax on earnings to be deferred into the future (ie, life insurance policies).
- Tax qualified products: investment funds such as retirement plans that allow monies to be invested before paying income taxes on them.

Reinvest Back Into Your Rehab Business

Besides all of the tax and accumulation benefits that have been mentioned, there is one more lesson to be remembered at all times: The best return you will ever make is back into your own business.

Here is some good advice:

- Continue to be passionate and motivated about how to improve your own skills as a professional, as well as the skills of your employees. Employees that are made to feel appreciated and attended to generally work harder and better and are loyal to your rehab business' objectives. Provide productivity incentives, make additions to benefits packages, and give money allowances for educational seminars and courses that will directly affect the quality of client care.
- Delegate non–client-related tasks to office personnel to free up your time to allow marketing and networking with existing clients, referral sources, and payers. Your personal attention will keep the business flowing and the marketing objectives met.
- Upgrade expense items to facilitate your rehab business image, integrity, and position among your competitors (eg, leasing or purchasing new pediatric therapy equipment that provides alternative, innovative interventions for sensory integration treatment).
- Upgrade your operating office systems to conduct efficient office tasks such as medical billing, scheduling, and other related tasks that are time-consuming with older office systems.

✛ *Manage Your Risks*

Think of the ways you are exposed to any personal liability and may suffer personal losses. This process will generally allow you to identify the financial risks that you may be exposed to just by being in business.

Here are some financial risks that you can manage:

- Avoid unintentional long-term agreements or business decisions that obligate your business revenues or have a greater impact than it can withstand, such as leasing more rental space than you need or can afford.
- Avoid overspending on start-up costs and operating costs that can be purchased at a later time or as needed. Spend your money and time on the basic essentials.
- Avoid overspending on payrolls by investigating and paying competitive, but reasonable, salary rates.

Special Considerations for the Rehab Professional

Increasing your profitability and managing risks require that you learn how to examine some key operating items.[4] Monitoring your numbers is vital to reducing your operating budget expenses.

- Net sales: Compare gross revenue minus third-party payer contractual allowances. Generally, rehab businesses receive 40% of the total dollars charged in contractual allowances.
- Professional payroll: This percentage number depends on productivity standards, but generally 15% of net revenue is spent on payroll (lower if fewer staff).
- Office payroll: This typically comes to 14% of net revenue.
- Overhead expenses: This includes renting space and, on average, consumes 20% of net revenue.
- Indirect expenses: Items like marketing, legal fees, and accounting can account for 7% of your net revenue.

STEP 4: UNDERSTAND THE BASICS TO BILLING AND REIMBURSEMENT

In Chapter 5, you learned about four areas of reimbursement that require further learning: sources of payment, payment methodologies, billing and coding, and provider networks. Here we will cover the basics. If you decide to perform your own billing and collecting, we recommend that you seek further learning by participating in industry or payer-specific educational opportunities. Both AOTA and APTA include learning courses or seminars through their website, conferences, or products. Secondly, network with area colleagues who are presently owners to gain personal advice and recommendations in regard to reimbursement. Billing and collecting is complicated and time consuming. If done incorrectly, you could jeopardize your hard work and best intentions.

Determine Sources of Income

Understanding basic accounting is the fundamental component of financial responsibility that provides the basic skills needed for billing and collecting. Next, you will need to determine how you will get paid for your services.

There are three major options:

1. Private pay (cash)
2. Insurance
3. Charities/Foundations/Grants/Donations

Private pay is the easiest for you, but it is traditionally not the way clients are accustomed to paying for health care services. Although, clients are familiar with receiving an invoice sent to them from the practitioner with a sum owed after their insurance has made payment on their account. Private pay can be cash, check, credit card, gift cards, or any other type of monetary payment that is not associated with insurance. Have your accounting system and banking system set up to take credit cards and automatic deposits to avoid heavy reliance on personal checks, which come with a greater payment risk.

Pricing therapy for private pay should be "UCR" (usual, customary, and reasonable) for your geographic area. Medicare fees are generally thought of as the UCR to begin determining your private pay fees. You can obtain current pricing by visiting www.cms.hhs.gov and submitting a treatment code along with your area code. This will bring up a typical amount of reimbursement. Keep that in mind, then attempt to determine your overhead costs for running your practice using those fixed and variable numbers that you just learned about. Take your monthly cost of operations and divide down to an hourly amount of overhead cost.

You now have two numbers to guide you: the typical fee amount you could expect from Medicare for an hour of therapy, and the cost of performing that work in your practice. You will determine a UCR pricing based on your decision of meeting overhead, UCR, and making a net profit. Utilize your experts such as an accountant, medical biller, and colleagues to gauge your decision.

Example:

60 minutes of therapy	=	[97110 (therapeutic exercise) x 2 units (each $32.44)]
		+ [97112(neuromuscular reeducation) x 1 unit ($34.06)]
		+ [97535(self care/home management) x 1 unit ($35.05)]
	=	$133.33
Hourly overhead expenses	=	total monthly expenses ÷ total billable hours (direct client contact)
	=	$74.00 per hour
		Your net is $59.33 (45%).

Therefore, your starting fees per service should be in a range between $60 to $192 per hour just to either break even or make a typical net profit overall.

Insurance can be divided into two main categories for the sake of convenience: commercial insurance companies and federal and state insurance programs. Commercial insurance can be further defined as managed care organizations, while federal and state insurance programs are generally Medicare and Medi-cal/Medi-caid and derivatives of those.

Managed care organizations are network-based corporations that provide health care coverage by levels of service providers and pre-determined financial methodologies. They can be broken down into these main types:

- Health maintenance organizations (HMO)
  o Members have primary care physicians who determine service needs.
  o Services require prior authorization and are within a contracted network of providers.
  o Copayment for services is taken at the time of service and deducted from reimbursement.
- Preferred Provider Organization (PPO)
  o Member has choice of physicians and providers.
  o Reimbursement is based on a fee schedule discount.
  o Members have a deductible and a coinsurance.
- Point of service (POS)
  o Members are similar to PPO, but plans have higher costs to patients.
  o Members can go out of network but will pay more for services out of their pockets.
  o Payments vary according to usage and specialty.
- Independent Practice Assocations (IPA)
  o Functions like HMOs with a capitation-based payment.
- Indemnity insurance plans
  o Members are reimbursed for their out-of-pocket health care services based on plan policies.

The reimbursement for your services is therefore generally determined by the insurance policy of your clients. If you decide to participate in these insurance programs, you will need to have a contract with the carrier. In some cases, like for those plans that do not require "in-network" relationships, you will need to call the carrier to obtain necessary information to perform the coding and/or billing process. In addition, some carriers require that you submit "credentialing" applications for your practice and each of your employee therapists. Many of them also require copies of your license, NPI number, articles of incorporation, leases, and other types of small business documents to satisfy their requirements for payment.

Medicare and Medi-caid/Medi-cal are federal and state insurance programs that require a provider enrollment process that ends with obtaining a PTAN (provider transaction access number) for your practice and you as an individual. If you have employees, you may also have to submit additional paperwork on their behalf in order for them to perform services to your clients. Members of federal and state insurance programs have met specific criteria and, like commercial insurance programs, have to obtain services from credentialed providers. Reimbursement is determined by established regional rates per billing code and time, and it requires specific billing forms and processing methodology. Obtaining assistance through your state or national therapy association or by hiring a knowledgeable medical billing company is a must. There can be penalties and fines for incorrectly billed services.

If you are a nonprofit business model, then you will be receiving your monies from your relationship with a charity, foundation, or other type of donations. As was mentioned in Chapter 2, monies allocated for services is usually defined within your business plan and operating budget. Generally, the clients or participants are receiving services pro bono or by organizational "scholarship." You are being paid by a contractual amount predetermined by budget. The financial responsibility is more of an accounting task and not a collections task.

Implement Necessary Reimbursement Documents

Regardless of your source of income or reimbursement, there are necessary documents that need to be in place. Documentation compliance will be different from state to state depending on the type of payer and by state regulations and licensure. Those include but are not limited to:

- Intake form
- HIPAA privacy statement
- Verification of benefits/Authorization
- Explanation of benefits
- Prescription
- Evaluation or assessment
- Treatment plan or Plan of Care (POC)
- Progress notes
- Discharge summary
- Charge slips/superbill
- Specific billing forms such as HCFA 1500

The content of your documentation is important in order to limit reimbursement denials, restrictions, or delays if you are billing insurance programs. The general rules of engagement include:

- To be covered, therapy must be reasonable and necessary.
- Therapy must be ordered by a physician.
- The patient's condition and level of complexity require the skills of a qualified therapist.
- The medical record contains documentation with measurable and functional goals.
- Therapy is provided by a certified therapist or by a licensed provider supervised by the certified therapist.
- Therapy must be provided with the expectation that the patient's condition will improve in a reasonable period of time.
- Therapy will only be covered as long as documentation supports the improvement of the patient.
- Therapy will be covered according to insurance policy.

If you are taking private pay clients only, then the rule of thumb is to follow any documentation requirements given in your state licensure and regulations or any other oversight agency. Nonprofit business models are often asked to include assessments (pre- and post-) and general treatment note writing with applicable and outcome measurements.

Identify Guidelines to Coding and Billing

If you have decided to establish contractual relationships to third party payers such as the insurance programs, then you will have to learn how to code and bill for services. You will learn the very basics here to get you started, but additional learning or expert assistance is essential. There are diagnostic codes and procedural codes. The diagnostic codes (ICD –9-CM) represent the exact acute problem you are evaluating for treatment. They can be found in print or online at www.medical-coding.net. Generally speaking, the client will come to you with a prescription with a diagnosis indicated by the treating physician. The diagnosis has at least a 4-digit code (ie, ACL repair 844.2) associated with it, similar to the idea of a bar code representing a specific retail item. Procedural codes (CPT) are 5-digit numbers that represent your specific treatment intervention or modality such as therapeutic activities (97530) or ultrasound (97035). They are timed or not timed in 15 to 30 minute increments. Splints and other supplies also have codes assigned to them. In summary, an hour of therapeutic intervention is represented by several codes, which are indicated on a super-bill or specific billing form and submitted electronically to a clearinghouse. The clearinghouse then directs them to the specific insurance carrier who processes the billing and sends you and the client an explanation of benefits (EOB) with a reimbursement check or payment.

Managed care plans such as HMOs have capitated rates and often tell you which code they want you to submit on the billing form in order to comply with their processing. For example, the insurance company may have a contract that states the code they will accept is therapeutic exercises (97110) for 30 minutes to be billed at $40 minus the copayment. If you have a contracted relationship with the carrier, then this is exactly how you will bill.

Medicare, on the other hand, allows you to code and bill for services rendered within the time indicated by you. They will reimburse you according to UCR in your geographical area and within their specific guidelines of medical necessity, supervision, timed and not timed codes, and so forth. Both AOTA and APTA offer valuable information and links to the Centers for Medicare and Medicaid Services for further learning.

Most importantly, make sure your documentation supports your intervention, which, in turn, supports your billing codes, which, in turn, complies with your contract or with the reimbursement methodology of the payer. The most common reasons for denial are:

- Unable to determine medical necessity
- Overall inadequate documentation
- Client shows no significant improvement within a reasonable and predictable time period
- Duplication of services
- Truncated or incorrect diagnosis code
- No current prescription

You will need to purchase billing software in order to produce and send the billing forms required. There are many to chose from. Go to the buyer's guide at such publications as www.rehabpub.com or AOTA or APTA practice journals to obtain the names and websites of billing software. Some software programs are built for larger organizations, so make sure you are selecting a product that fits your needs.

Financial management is critical to any business. Business success depends on how well you bring your product or service to the customer in a cost-effective strategy. Your business has to be perceived as providing a real benefit to the customer that he or she cannot do for him- or herself at your price. Armed with this information, you can begin to formulate your business development model while answering the following questions:

- How much capital will it take to initiate the start-up of my business? $ _____
- What are the purchase expenses that I must make to begin services? $ _____
- How much money do I need to have for living expenses for the first year? $ _____
- What do I absolutely have to have now, and what could be purchased on an as-needed basis?

_____

- What are the fixed expenses that must happen now?

_____

- What are the variable expenses that I must incur now?

_____

- How much cash flow will it take to cover those expenses as they come due? $ _____
- How much of my product or service must I produce on a weekly basis to cover the above expense items?
          $ _____
- In a perfect world, how much product or service must I produce to reach positive cash flow, break even, and finally, profitability?

_____

- How am I going to be paid for my services?

_____

- Do I have the skills to perform the billing of my services, or should I hire a medical billing company?

_____

- Do I and my employee practitioners have the documentation skills and knowledge needed to support the billing codes and any request for information?

_____

Tips and Tools

It is not reasonable to expect that you will be paid timely or without denials or requests for additional information such as copies of your documentation.

Here are some tips to dealing with common denials or requests:

- Implement evidence-based practice or standards of practice when able to. Send in copies of your evidence-based research or "evidence briefs" to support your intervention that may be in question.

- Know and have a copy of your licensure or regulations. It is common to receive a statement from the carrier that they feel you are working outside of your scope of practice. You will need to educate them on your scope of practice by sending them a copy and highlighting the areas that support your services.

- Implement outcome measurements (either formal or informal) such as pain level, formal pre- and post-assessments, or even patient satisfaction surveys. Send copies of your outcome measurements if questioned about the patient's progress or medical necessity.

- Make sure to perform your progress notes every two weeks or once a month. This documentation shows functional gains and improvements to support additional visits.

- Always give the client a home management program, and make sure to keep a copy of it in the medical chart. Insurance carriers want to know that you are advocating for client responsibility of healing and proactive discharge from services.

- Reevaluate clients when gains have been made and record measurements. Objective measurements are more powerful than subjective words when fighting for reimbursement.

For nonprofit organizations, make sure you are asking the administrator of the grant or charity for any specific documentation such as what pre-/post-assessments or outcome measurements are expected of the grant, and better yet, what type of goals they are hoping to reach that are representative of the grant they want to go after. For example, some grants will clearly state that they support programs that prevent falling. Therefore, you would have to make sure you can measure balance and falling, and have or will implement the necessary tools.

CHAPTER 6 SUMMARY

Step 1: Understand Accounting Basics
- Complete the following accounting tasks:
  - ❒ Hire an accountant.
  - ❒ Purchase accounting software or develop a bookkeeping system.
  - ❒ Obtain a business checking account and business credit card.
  - ❒ Develop a method of tracking business receipts.
  - ❒ Organize your financial statements.
  - ❒ Perform regular bookkeeping activities.

Step 2: Manage Your Cash Flow
  - ❒ Create a cash flow projection statement (see Chapter 3) with your specific fixed and variable expense items.
  - ❒ Organize and file all contractual agreements for real estate leases, equipment leases, purchase agreements, sales agreements, and related documents.

Step 3: Improve Your Profitability and Manage Your Risks
  - ❒ Once your rehab business is up and running, go back and examine the several avenues available to you for improving your cash flow on a regular basis.
  - ❒ Manage your risks by keeping several decision-making and operating concepts in mind.

Step 4: Understand the Basics to Coding and Billing
  - ❒ Determine your income sources, and remember that you can take cash and insurance.
  - ❒ Implement necessary documents and contracts.
  - ❒ Purchase and implement billing software.
  - ❒ Obtain further knowledge and skills or hire a medical billing company.

Action Plan
  - ❒ Learn accounting, coding, and billing basics by attending seminars, courses, and classes.
  - ❒ Hire professional help.

References

1. Internal Revenue Service. Publication 583: starting a business and keeping records. Available at: http://www.irs.gov/pub/irs-pdf/p583.pdf. Accessed March 26, 2004.

2. All Business. Finance and accounting center. Available at: http://www.allbusiness.com/accounting/2984839-1.html. Accessed December 30, 2008.

3. Keller J. Money matters: max out your receivable with 14 simple steps. *Advance for Directors in Rehabilitation* [serial online]. 2002;11(4):11. Available at: http://rehabilitation-director.advanceweb.com/Editorial/Search/AViewer.aspx?AN=DR_02apr1_drp11.html&AD=04-01-2002. Accessed October 30, 2008.

4. Guihan L, Klos C. Cash flow. *Advance for Directors in Rehabilitation* [serial online]. 2002;11(3):15-16. Available at: http://rehabilitation-director.advanceweb.com/Editorial/Search/AViewer.aspx?AN=DR_02mar1_drp15.html&AD=03-01-2002. Accessed October 30, 2008.

Suggested Reading

Ensman R Jr. Money matters: is it time to switch from a cash-based to an accrual accounting system? *Advance for Directors in Rehabilitation*. 2007;16(9):16-17.

Internal Revenue Service. Publication 535: business expenses. Available at: http://www.irs.gov/pub/irs-pdf/p535.pdf. Accessed March 26, 2004.

Internal Revenue Service. Publication 552: recordkeeping for individuals. Available at: http://www.irs.gov/pub/irs-pdf/p552.pdf. Accessed March 26, 2004.

Jordan C. Is it time to tame the cash flow problem? *Advance for Directors in Rehabilitation*. 2007;16(10):15-16.

Le Postollec M. Money lenders: business-savvy private practitioners can use loans to launch their clinics. *Advance for Directors in Rehabilitation*. 2001;10(11):15-16.

Nolo. Business income defined. Available at: http://www.nolo.com/lawcenter/ency/article.cfm/ObjectID/97A1F3ED-BD41-42A5-88617BAF3DD299C8/catID/AC0056C4-8316-4E15-B230718361C43BEA. Accessed April 17, 2003.

Nosse L, Friberg D, Kovacek P. *Managerial and Supervisory Principles for Physical Therapists*. Philadelphia, PA: Williams & Wilkens; 1999.

Palacio M. 25 secrets of profitability in private practice. *Online Advance for Occupational Therapy Practitioners* [serial online]. 2000. Available at: http://occupational-therapy.advanceweb.com/Editorial/Search/AViewer.aspx?CC=7559. Accessed October 30, 2008.

Pinson L, Jinnett J. *Steps to Small Business Start-Up*. 4th ed. Chicago, IL: Dearborn; 2000.

Electronic Resources

www.irs.gov: Internal Revenue Service; Information for businesses, charities, and nonprofit organizations; forms; and publications.

www.medical-coding.net: Medical coding website for products and learning.

www.accuchecker.com: Health care reimbursement website.

REFLECT AND REDIRECT

Beverly Sumwalt, MT (ASCP), MA

Tammy Richmond, MS, OTRL

Beverly Sumwalt, MT (ASCP), MA

Tammy Richmond, MS, OTRL

CHAPTER OBJECTIVES

✓ Reflect on performance and productivity.
✓ Redirect to enhance profit and reduce expenses.

*"The difference between success and failure is directly proportional
to the distance between vision and action."*
B. Sumwalt

Congratulations, your new business is off and running! You have created your business with your vision and mission in mind, built a solid business structure, and developed and implemented strong business and marketing plans. Now it is time for a little "R&R"—Reflect and Redirect.

Any good plan is dynamic (ie, it is constantly changing, capitalizing on new opportunities, eliminating inefficiencies, and growing or downsizing to suit the market). Good businesses rely on constant monitoring, ongoing feedback, and assessment of "how are we doing?" in order to keep the focus on growth, productivity, and of course, profitability. There are two key steps in this feedback loop that are mandatory for continued success:

Step 1: Reflect on performance and productivity.

Step 2: Redirect to enhance profit and reduce expenses.

As you begin these steps, you will need to combine all of the skills you have learned in Chapters 1 through 6 and bring them together to help you with the assessment of your business, and then with the implementation of any modifications you choose to make based on the assessment. There may be only two steps to this part of your business, but in several ways, they are the most important ones!

STEP 1: REFLECT ON PERFORMANCE AND PRODUCTIVITY

The word reflect is defined as "to give back an image, a mirror" and "to contemplate or ponder."[1] To reflect on your business is to look at it as others see it and to think carefully about how it is operating. Completing a business performance assessment does this effectively and systematically.

The five main elements of such an assessment include:
1.   Revisit your vision and mission statements.
2.   Review your business plan.
3.   Revitalize the marketing plan.
4.   Review the financials and return on investment (ROI).
5.   Reevaluate the implementation plan.

You have written your business plan, formulating the infrastructure on the basis of your vision, your mission, your services and values, and your market. Now that you have been using that plan, the answers to those tough questions will be more clear than when you were doing the original assessments. You know more and you have some metric data to support the conclusions that you made assumptions about in the early stages of your rehab business concept. Let's take it through the process again, this time with more experience and information.

✛ Revisit Your Vision and Mission Statements

Have any of your personal or professional goals changed? Is the list of services you provide still the same? Read your vision statement—are you still inspired? Read your mission statement—are you still directed? If so, then you're on the right track and ready to continue. If they seem "off" to you, make notes and continue on. If your vision and mission have changed, you will need to make adjustments accordingly when we move to Step 2 of this process.

✛ Review Your Business Plan

In Chapters 1, 2, and 3, you carefully charted your business opportunities, set up your organizational structure, wrote out a detailed document demonstrating all of the parameters that would contribute to your success, and identified those threats that could be contributors to failure. Read through your business plan again. If you were thorough and complete with this process in the initial phase, you will be pleased to see how clearly it defines what is actually happening. Bankers and investors who make their living by choosing and supporting successful business plans will tell you that little changes over time with the initial plan—what changes is the strategy a company uses to implement the plan. As you read, make notes of any changes, new or revised information, or creative ideas that come into play. Now that you have some experience behind you, it is easy to see how it all fits together just like you planned it.

✛ Revitalize the Marketing Plan

In Chapter 4, you learned all of the components that make up a dynamic marketing plan. As you read your plan again, ask these questions:

- Has the industry changed? Perform a SWOT analysis on your current operations and marketing plan to see where the changes have taken place. Visit the websites of state and national associations and read up on the emerging trends and current practice areas to compare your findings with the overall bigger picture of your industry.

- Are there trends, new techniques, or technologies that impact your services that did not exist when this plan was written? Create a client satisfaction and new service questionnaire to see what services they are interested in and how you are doing with your present services. Continue to scan newspapers, articles, and online social networks to get a sense of trends, societal demands, and useful technologies that you may want to incorporate to reach more people. There are new software or web programs developed to "push" your message to your audience such as email alerts and social site logo advertisements.

- Has your target market or the demographics of your service area changed? Have you noticed that your referral sources have been sending you more or less of a certain population type or type of diagnosis? Has there been a change in your surrounding physical environment such as new businesses in the area that are attracting a different age group or economical group that may impact your choice of marketing strategies? Maybe it's time to go back out and make drop-by visits to these new businesses to pass out flyers and business cards, or to set up meetings with the managers or owners to introduce your practice and to hear about the particular needs of their employees and client base.

- Is the collateral material outdated? Does your printed marketing material look fresh, contain your current list of services, and reflect changes in your internal or external environments. Maybe you just added some new equipment and changed the layout of your space. Your marketing materials should reflect your "newly-remodeled and state-of-the-art equipment" changes.

- Are your promotional strategies still appropriate? It's easy to become relaxed about your community outreach efforts and personal selling when your business is going well. Maybe it's time to re-energize your marketing efforts by first reflecting on your current marketing plan, asking for feedback from your staff, and coming up with some new marketing tasks that utilize both your staff and your current clients and referral sources. For example, set up a lunch-and-learn lecture of "new treatments and emerging services in Parkinson's Disease," and invite your referring physician, medical vendor, and your staff to present and demonstrate new information and services to your present and potential clients.

This part of the "reflect" is where you will undoubtedly find things to change. Now that you've been in business for a while, you have a better feel for your market, your clients and referral sources, your vendors, and your marketing impact, and you should see several things that you already know you want to change. You should also have data to back up your intuition and support you in making the right amount of change. Overcorrecting things can sometimes be worse than not changing them at all, so use your data as your guide. Spend plenty of time with your marketing plan because the notes you make here will be your building blocks as you move to "redirect" things in Step 2.

✛ *Review the Financials and Return on Investments*

Your financial picture will tell you a lot about your success so far. Gather together your monthly financial statements, your bank statements, and your checkbook, and let's see how the "picture" looks. Your monthly accounting should reflect revenues and expenses, and your bank statements, deposits, and withdrawals should match accordingly.

It is not the intent in this chapter to give financial management guidelines, but rather to define how the financial picture reflects on how the business is doing. Here, you want to look at expenses and see if they tend to support your services.

Ask yourself these questions:

- Are they in line with what you're actually doing?

- Does anything stand out as a large expense that doesn't have a correspondingly large revenue source? If so, that is something to note for change or "redirection." Check out the office and medical supplies expense total. This is a common place for overspending and waste.

- Look at your cash flow and note where the largest revenue streams come from. Are there any threats, trends, etc that could affect large revenue sources and suddenly upset the financial picture? This is where going back to your external threats (eg, changes in the reimbursement environment or changes to your state licensure and regulations) is vital. For example, the Medicare cap and quarterly changes to Medicare guidelines and reimbursement is a direct and important impact to a practice that services that population and gets paid by Medicare monies. You may need to consider refocusing your marketing efforts on another population that has dropped off such as commercial payers, or expand your menu of services to include cash services such as yoga or Pilates classes.

- Are there revenues that are steady versus intermittent, and how do they affect the cash flow of the business?

- Do the revenue sources match up with the expense items? Are you and your staff taking advantage of the new piece of equipment you purchased, or it is time for another staff training session to raise awareness of the benefits and treatment goals of the modality?

- If you employ staff, do your payroll expenses reasonably match up with increases in business revenues? Can you cross-train your staff to perform several internal business roles or job responsibilities so you can reduce your dependency on per diem staff and/or contracted outside vendors?

- What is your ROI? Basically, what is your net income overall or with a specific service, product, or program. ROI is that bottom line number showing how much profit is made compared to how much was spent. For example, you buy a new treadmill and invested X dollars. You are making Y dollars from treadmill appointments. If Y is greater than X, your ROI is positive (and vice versa). This is a number that will be of interest to your investors, your banker, and your tax accountant.

Again, this is not an attempt to give financial advice, but a reasonable assumption is that if you invest some money in your business, you should expect a reasonable return profit on that investment. Externally, it means the business is profitable and you get to keep some of that profit. Internally, it means that each and every business decision you make that requires you to spend money should result in revenue being generated. The old adage of "you have to spend money to make money" is very true, so when you review your financial picture, make sure the decisions you have been making to spend money are demonstrating good financial return. Notes here are critical and will help you make tough decisions in the marketing and staffing areas as you redirect your resources.

✛ Reevaluate the Implementation Plan

Undoubtedly, as you worked through the set up and configuration of your business, not everything went like clockwork. Now it is time to look at those hard assets, the policies and procedures, the management issues, and the contracts that bring it all together. We refer to all of that as "operations." Essentially, it's the infrastructure that allows you to implement your action plans.

Operations Reevaluation

- Is your space sufficient, or do you need to add or reduce your facility space? Maybe it is time to move things around to take advantage of the outlets, windows, and corners.
- Do you have adequate parking and equipment? Is the equipment you have being utilized to capacity?
- Are there better uses of space now that you see how the workflow is accomplished? Take a walk around your facility, inside and outside, and let your eyes see it as one of your clients would. Do some areas look messy and chaotic? Are entrances and exits pleasing?
- At your busiest time, is parking available, and could a handicapped person find his or her way easily?
- Does your treatment space feel crowded, empty and vacuous, or "just right" and efficient?
- Is your administrative space cluttered or neat and efficient? Is there enough dedicated space for effective documentation, charts, and supplies? Time is money, and money is lost when your space becomes disorganized. Set aside "spring cleaning" and "fall clean-out" as your time for everyone to get reacquainted with what's being used and what is being overlooked or misplaced.

These are indicators of how your facility is seen by others, and it also gives you valuable clues about whether you are using your space in the most efficient and effective way. Space is expensive, so make notes here about revising the way it looks or serves you and your clients. As part of your "walkthrough," you will also want to assess your capital equipment and how it is performing for you. When you did your financial assessment, you would have noted lease or loan payments for equipment and/or purchases, and compared them to revenues generated. Now look and see if there are things you need to replace, remove, or repair so that they are being used effectively.

Documentation Assessment

- Are your employment policies and procedures in place and up to date? Has everyone read the updates and initialed the pages?
- Do you have personnel records, contract files, and medical records all in a secure and locked space? Are you meeting HIPAA requirements?
- If you employ staff, are training and in-service schedules current? Do you have risk guidelines and labor relations issues posted? The personnel files need to contain copies of your professional license, memberships to industry associations, copies of your professional development units or continued educational units, employee or contractor agreements, and a yearly professional background check (you should be able to do this online through your licensure board website).
- In short, are your administrative functions working smoothly, or are they taking too much of your time away from revenue-generating functions?
- Are there any functions you can delegate or outsource that can be financially justified? Maybe you need to upgrade your software to make reconciling accounts and tracking specific business parameters easier.

Make a list of all of those things that you really hate to do (now that you have had some practice doing them) or of things that have ended back on your plate, and see whether it might be cost-effective to outsource them or delegate them to a staff member whose time you are already paying for. For example, the front office receptionist is generally also capable of filing, making call backs, marketing, ordering supplies, faxing, and several other back office tasks.

In reevaluating your operations, be sure you review all of your contracts and agreements. Look for outdates, automatic increases in fees, and decreases in reimbursements you may have forgotten. Assess whether some should be terminated or renegotiated, or if some fees could be lowered now that you have a business track record (this applies to things like legal retainers, accounting services, etc, where utilization has now been established and you do have the necessary "start-up advice or accounting templates" etc, so retainer fees or monthly service fees could potentially be reduced).

Use the Business Performance Assessment on p. 138 to help you with Step 1.

Tips and Tools

To assist you with reflecting and assessment:

- Have your accountant provide you with a summary financial statement (income statement), trend report, and current balance sheet.
- Ask your legal advisor, AOTA, APTA, or state organizations for an update on health care laws and hot issues that could affect your business.
- Pull your original market research data and spot-check it for accuracy in the present market environment.
- Consider the unbiased opinion and recommendations of a business analyst or small business consultant.

Most colleges/junior colleges offer business consultation as part of their business school services. There are also numerous Senior Retired Executives organizations that advise, consult, and serve small business entrepreneurs in their communities. For a nominal fee, you could pull together your vision and mission statements, business and marketing plans, and financial trend report, and have an expert review your business. You could also ask for an "on-site" assessment. This valuable service has several advantages:

- They are usually very inexpensive for very high-powered expertise.
- It is an unbiased snapshot assessment of your business and services.
- You can choose whether to act on recommendations without obligation or commitment to services.

This exercise is designed to help you assemble the information necessary to take the next step in the process, and to better define the next level of growth and development for your business.

STEP 2: REDIRECT TO ENHANCE PROFIT AND REDUCE EXPENSES

We all "redirect" things, alter our courses, and make new choices and decisions as our businesses grow and expand. The important thing is to know when you are "redirecting" and not just "reacting." Redirection is done with purpose, with supportive information, and with the goal of either enhancing profitability or reducing expenses. Reacting is usually done in crisis mode and rarely solves problems or creates long-lasting solutions. Your list for possible redirection will be derived from Step 1, during the reflection process.

As you choose things for redirection, ask yourself two important questions:
- Will it enhance profitability?
- Will it reduce expenses?

If the answer to either one is "yes," then you are on solid ground to proceed. If the answer to both is "no," then you should make that redirection a priority.

Redirection will be a direct result of evaluating (ie, reflecting on) your business and will most likely occur in the operational areas, including:
- Outreach and marketing plan
- Facility design and utilization
- Staffing and contracted services
- Accounting and legal retaining fees
- Fee schedules and reimbursement contracts
- Menu of services offered

Business Performance Assessment

Vision Statement
- Revisions needed: _____
_____
_____
_____

Mission Statement
- Revisions needed: _____
_____
_____
_____

Business Plan
- Revisions needed: _____
_____
_____
_____

Marketing Plan
- Revisions needed: _____
_____
_____
_____

Financials
- Revisions needed: _____
_____
_____
_____

Implementation
- Operations revisions: _____
_____
_____
_____

- Documentation revisions: _____
_____
_____
_____

Miscellaneous notes:
_____
_____
_____

✛ Outreach and Marketing Plan

Marketing can be a "high cost, low return" function if you do it without studying the results. In Chapter 4, you learned how to put together a comprehensive marketing plan, and you learned about the five P's of marketing assessment and analysis.

Now that you have business history to compare with your original marketing plan, ask yourself the following questions:

- *Where does my business come from?* "How did you hear about us?" is one of the best questions you can ask your customers. Then, use that to adjust your marketing budget and where you spend your money (redirecting expenditures to enhance profits).

- *Are my collateral materials inviting and informative?* Review them, ask the opinion of some of your steady clients, and see if your flyers, brochures, and business advertisements could be reduced in number, put out for rebid (reducing expenses), or distributed to a wider audience (enhancing profits).

- *Are we targeting the right places to distribute marketing collateral?* Should we have brochures at the local senior center since we have had no business from them in the last year, or should we step up our outreach to them (could be enhanced profits or reduced expenses depending on your "redirection")?

✛ Facility Design and Utilization

Your physical plant is your "showroom." We all get overly accustomed to our work environments. After a while, we do not see the ding in the bathroom wall, the frayed chair in the waiting room, or even worse—the cartoons and sayings plastered all over the workspace walls! Some are merely "cleanup" items, and some require expenditure to repair or replace. However, you want to balance expenditures for the space with whether it will enhance either your ability to deliver quality service or the appearance of your ability to deliver quality service.

Ask yourself the following questions:

- *Is the space adequate for the service my business delivers?* If not, you will need to consider increasing the space (expense). However, you must evaluate whether you will be able to perform the increased services to pay for the space (enhanced profits). A cost/benefit analysis is the only way to answer this question, and it should be performed before you remodel, lease, or build additional space. Opinions vary on when you should expect a positive return on your investment, but if the expenditure does not break even on cost/benefit analysis at its inception, you should strongly consider other alternatives before expansion.

- *Can the space be utilized more efficiently?* Consider expanding hours (customer service, enhancing profits). Perhaps procedures or services can be redirected to specific time slots, thus keeping all of the space productive rather than having procedure rooms empty (enhancing profit). Perhaps services can be delivered "offsite" (as in the local senior center), which would increase visibility and outreach to the community (enhancing profits) and could postpone or avoid the need to build another treatment room (reducing expense). Have your receptionist keep a log of the number of people in your waiting room every half hour during business hours. Is the space over- or underutilized? Is there room to put out products that you sell (enhancing profits)? Could you partition off part of it and use it for an administrative function, thereby opening up procedure space (enhancing profits)? Can you sublease to the office next door to share waiting room space and share reception costs (reducing expenses)?

✛ Staffing and Contracted Services

Labor costs are your highest overhead, and your most valuable asset. Using staff efficiently and outsourcing where appropriate is very critical to good business profitability. Ask yourself:

- *Have I done a recent human resource survey to determine salary standards for my area?* Are you able to hire new or additional staff at competitive rates (reducing expenses) and offer reduced hours or flex time to more expensive staff (reducing expenses)? Administratively, can you outsource payroll and benefits to an employee leasing company (employee enhancement, which reduces turn-over, which reduces expenses and enhances profitability)?

- *Is my staff productive during their paid time?* Can you delegate additional tasks rather than hire additional people (enhancing profits)? Can you adjust staffing patterns to increase the number of procedures that can be scheduled or allow you to offer expended hours (enhancing profits)? Do you have the "right person in the right job," paying only for the expertise needed? For example, you don't need a licensed professional doing administrative functions—hire a receptionist and reduce the hours of the licensed personnel (reducing expenses).

✢ Accounting and Legal Retaining Fees

As mentioned in Step 1, you have different needs in the start-up phase than you do in a more mature business. You may likely have both an accountant and a lawyer on retainer, which in start-up is more expensive because you must call them often. Now, it's likely you don't have to incur consultative time often.

Ask yourself:

- *Do I have any professional advice arrangements on retainer?* If yes, renegotiate the retainer based on the revised amount of time you need their services (reducing expenses). If no, this may not apply to your business.

- *Am I paying appropriate fees for retained or contracted professional services?* Do some shopping. Legal and accounting service fees vary widely, and you may find there are opportunities to lower the rates for both of these. If you find a better fee, go back to your advisors and ask for reduced rates (reducing expenses).

   [NOTE: This is not to advise you to "choose the cheapest service around town," but rather to advise you to shop wisely and get the best value for your money in professional services. Just going from retainers to hourly rates will be a move in the right direction now that you don't need daily advice.]

✢ Fee Schedules and Reimbursement Contracts

It is now time to take the information gained when you evaluated your fee schedules and contracts. Fee schedules are often set at the time you open doors for business, but then forgotten, and revisions may be necessary to be competitive. You may also have multiple contracts with health plans, medical groups, the local senior center, etc, and these should also be revisited for competitive advantage.

Ask yourself the following questions:

- *Do my fees reflect the current market fees for comparable services or procedures (enhancing revenue)?*

- *Does my fee schedule meet regulatory reimbursement legal guidelines (this could be expensive if not in compliance)?*

- *Do I need a "new and improved" fee schedule for my clients (customer service, enhancing revenue)?*

- *Are my contracts with health plans and all other payer entities up to date and current (enhancing revenue), and are they paying at the rate quoted?* You can always renegotiate your contract fees with a formal letter, with support letters from your referring sources and your patients, and with a general summary of what you offer, why it's more valuable and can reduce overall expenses and increase accessibility for the payer, what your patients and referring sources say about you, and how much you would like the increase to be. For example, several of you have advanced certifications or degrees or employ staff that have advanced degrees, yet you receive the same amount of reimbursement for an HMO policy. Does that seem fair? Of course not, so go back and renegotiate your rates based on the argument that there are several cost-effective benefits and patient benefits from your more expensive staff. Therefore, reimbursement should reflect your higher standards of care and services given.

   [NOTE: It is very wise to periodically compare your reimbursement statement codes with the quoted reimbursement rates in the contract, especially if you are doing capitated business. Many of the health plan contracts will change their reimbursement rates without notification, and all of a sudden you're receiving less revenue for your procedures (enhancing revenue).]

- *Should I cancel any contracts that are paying me less-than-acceptable rates (reducing expenses—poor reimbursement costs you money to administer with no return)?*

- *Should I seek more fee for service and/or less capitated business contracts (enhancing revenue)?*

✢ Menu of Services Offered

Your business enterprise has matured. As you reflect on the products and services you provide, there will no doubt be several new ideas you wish to put into your business implementation plan. You may wish to conduct a survey of your clients and referral sources, asking "What new services could we provide that you would be interested in?"

Ask yourself the following questions:

- *Am I providing the full scope of services to my clients, or could I add new services or procedures that now appear to be in demand (enhancing revenue)?* Conversely, do I have services or products that are not being utilized and should be dropped (reducing expenses)?

- *Are there support "products" that could be marketed in the office rather than sending clients to a device or product supplier (enhancing revenue)?* Should you consider expanding your present practice to include new programs and new personnel to perform those programs? Or, have you been asked to start a new program such as "fall prevention," so now you need to enhance your and your staff's skills and competencies to fulfill the demand?

- *Do client surveys indicate things that could be provided with high return on investment (enhancing revenue) and with little or no expenditure on staff or facilities (reducing expenses)?* This is a good time to evaluate offering services "offsite" (eg, to the local senior center, the local gym, an apartment complex in your area, and even the YMCA or rehab/skilled nursing facility). Offsite services are very popular and a good source of revenue with less expense than increasing facility space and capitalization (enhancing revenue). It's "free" marketing in it's own way (reducing expenses)!

- *Has my business explored some innovative thinking?* Have I asked my team what we might provide that would bring in more revenue, and that would be fun and interesting for them to participate in?

  [NOTE: Getting your staff involved with innovative "out-of-the-box" thinking can be very rewarding, provide job satisfaction for them, and give you creative new ways to improve your business (enhances revenue and reduces the expense of staff under-utilization and turnover)!]

Why do some businesses succeed and others fail? Much has been written about the success and failure of small businesses. This book has given you all of the tools used by the most successful businesses and entrepreneurs, and it paves a road to developing your own successful business. You now know the importance of the planning process and what you must do prior to seeing the first client to insure your business thrives. You also know how marketing affects the visibility and, ultimately, the profitability of your new young business. You are prepared for the financial commitment it takes to begin the venture and will not be surprised by the unexpected.

The following Business Success Flow Chart (see p. 142) may help you visualize how reflecting and redirecting will help you not only to maintain, but to grow and enhance your business.

Special Considerations for the Rehab Professional

Analyzing your business is a lot like assessing your clinical client. You gather both subjective and objective information about your business utilizing your staff, documentation, systems outcomes, and experts. Next, you determine the areas that are not performing as well or are costing you more than you expected or would like. Then, you direct your efforts into formulating a strategy plan, which is basically a smaller version of your business plan and more like your marketing action plan. Lastly, you implement the changes. In the business-sense, you are determining your "risks." Types of risk include physical, psychological, and financial.[2]

To start, gather the following items:

- ❏ Business Plan
- ❏ Marketing Plan and Marketing Materials
- ❏ Management and Operations Checklist
- ❏ Policy and Procedure Manual
- ❏ Employee Handbook
- ❏ Personnel Files
- ❏ Income Statement and Balance Statement
- ❏ Chart Reviews
- ❏ Aging Accounts Summary
- ❏ Vendor List
- ❏ Licensure Regulations; Scope of Practice
- ❏ Organizational Chart
- ❏ Insurance Policies

Examine your physical risks by making sure your insurance coverage is paid and adequate for your setting and your services. Call to see if there are any factors that would allow you to lower your premium costs. Check your policy and procedure manual, employee handbook, and personnel files to make sure they cover patient safety, equipment use and safety, OSHA guidelines, licensure regulations, labor laws such as breaks, lunches, time off, and other benefits, and that your staff has complied with the necessary amount of continued education units or professional development units. Medical equipment should be calibrated on a yearly basis, and every person working should be updated on use and protocols.

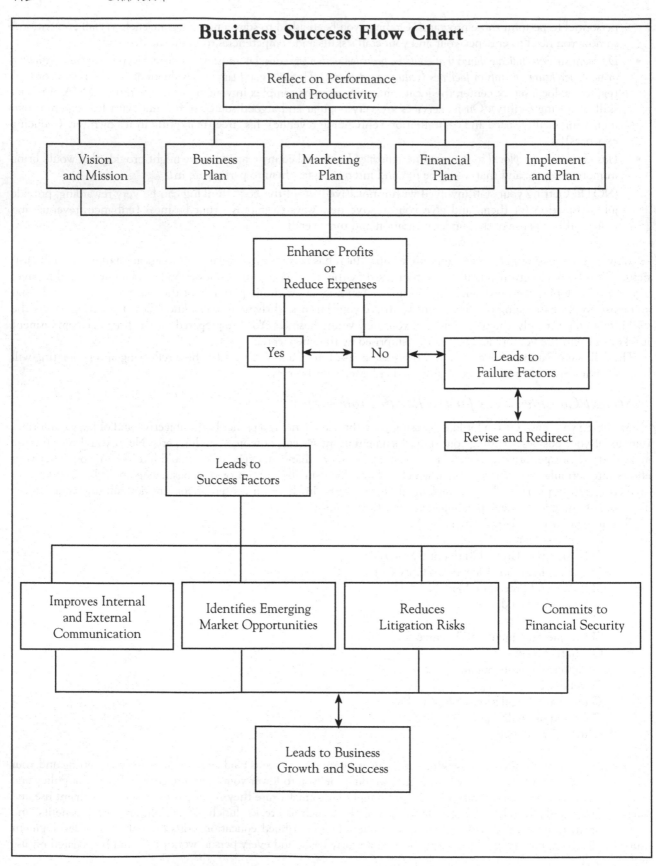

Examine your psychological risks by meeting with your staff and discussing non-billable time, down time, privacy issues, internal (personnel) issues, and to whom you have delegated tasks. Staff burnout, change in client flow over time, and just human behavior often become our silent-but-daunting risks. Make sure you are utilizing your staff and scheduling efficiently. Maybe you have the burnout and it's time that someone else does some of the operations or management tasks that can be completed by present staff or outsourced.

Allow an open, critique-welcomed session where folks can vent and you can listen. If you are a sole proprietor, find a mentor or colleague that you can confidentially go over matters with. Talking out loud can be so therapeutic and solution-getting. Client surveys or staff surveys also allow you important feedback about your services and how well management and operations are doing.

Examine your financial risk by pencil and paper and expert assistance. First, go over the expenses. Are there items like medical or office supplies that could be trimmed? Are you calling your various vendors and asking for free shipping and information on promotions that may save you money? Negotiate your interest on your business credit cards, and use credit cards that give you value-added services. Incidentals as simple as sending out invoices can add up, so see if your clients are open to receiving invoices by fax or email. Look at your non-billable services such as uncovered ultrasound treatments and heat/cold modalities, and make sure they are necessary in the treatment intervention. Items like hand putty and therapy balls are not generally covered, so you need to collect cash for those items from your clients. If you haven't already, collect all of your copayments at the time of service, and charge for last minute cancellations.

Next, you need to stay on top of billing claim denials, restrictions, and payments. Fee schedule and reimbursement methodologies used by carriers can change often. It is your responsibility to stay vigilant about your claims processing. Make sure your medical billing company or biller is accountable and on top of patient accounting. You should be performing at least quarterly chart reviews to make sure your documentation is legible, reflective of work performed, and clearly describing treatment in functional, measurable terms. If you are a cash business, make sure your charges accurately reflect your overhead costs. Furthermore, review your services, client volume, referral sources, and marketing materials. Maybe it's time to enhance your business with client-centered services or to create new, on-message marketing materials.

Assessing your financials takes time to go through the details, but it is worth every penny. And you are worth every penny. Don't give money away because you can't find the time to completely understand the dollars and sense!

CHAPTER 7 SUMMARY

Step 1: Reflect on Performance and Productivity

- Perform a Business Performance Assessment (see p. 138).

    ❑ Revisit your vision and mission statements. Rewrite them if necessary to currently reflect your personal and professional goals.

    ❑ Review the business plan. Rewrite those sections that need to be updated. The business plan acts as your résumé for your company, so it's always a good idea to update it.

    ❑ Revitalize the marketing plan. Eliminate those marketing strategies that did not bring in more patients or more money. Add marketing strategies that are more cost effective and have a proven track record. If you are still not meeting your business goals, then consider the value of social networking and community partnership.

    ❑ Review the financials and ROI. If you have hired an accountant, schedule quarterly phone meetings with him or her to go over the general accounting to see if there are any strategies available to cut costs and increase profits. Similarly, have regular weekly or at least bi-monthly discussions with your medical billing company or person. You should go over outstanding accounts receivables, denials, restrictions, or other limitations that are coming up during the billing and reimbursement process. Review any new federal-, state-, or insurance-imposed changes to reimbursement or documentation. Have a full understanding of the claims and billing process, and strategies to pursue outstanding monies.

    ❑ Reevaluate the implementation plan. You can go back and revisit Chapter 5 to review the implementation process. Again, utilize the Business Management and Operational Task list to double check that you are performing the necessary tasks to sustain your business and comply with regulations.

Step 2: Redirect to Enhance Profit and Reduce Expenses

As you redirect your business, you must always ask yourself:

- Is this enhancing profitability? Identify the specific areas—physical, psychological, or financial—that are costing you time and money and are not promoting profit or efficiency. _____

    _____

    _____

- Is this reducing expenses? Identify any specific areas, or use those you identified in question one, to create a strategy plan. Consult with experts, colleagues, and within yourself to write out the "how, what, where, when, and how much" answers to your problem areas. Spend the time and effort it takes to gather the necessary information to make sound business decisions now and not let business continue as usual if it is draining your energy and resources. Make sure to get your staff involved in the discussion. Often, they can add valuable information to the validity and needs of the business or how to run it more effectively or efficiently. Plus, you will need them to make the same emotional and physical commitments you are making in order to satisfy the patients, referral sources, and the payers.

You have successfully reflected on your business and all of the components that make it work, and have a new action plan for redirecting those things that make you money. This may well be the most important time you spend with your maturing business, and it should be done at regular intervals. The dynamics of the profession and the frequency of changes in the health care industry would suggest that business owners do this once every year, or even as soon as every six months. Now that you are familiar with the process, reflect and redirect with confidence!

Action Plan

    ❑ Perform a business performance assessment.

    ❑ Create a strategy plan with tasks and time tables to sustain your personal and business goals.

REFERENCES

1. *Webster's Dictionary*. 3rd college ed. New York, NY: Simon & Schuster, Inc; 1998:454.

2. Glinn J. Are you at risk? *Advance for Physical Therapists and PT Assistants* [serial online]. 2008;19(9):27. Available at: http://physical-therapy.advanceweb.com/Editorial/Search/AViewer.aspx?AN=PT_08apr21_ptp27.html&AD=04-21-2008. Accessed October 30, 2008.

SUGGESTED READING

Berry T. Kick-start your concept. Available at: http://articles.bplans.com/index.php/business-articles/starting-a-business/kick-start-your-concept/208. Accessed December 8, 2008.

Braveman B. *Leading & Managing Occupational Therapy Services: An Evidence-Based Approach*. Chicago, IL: F.A. Davis Company; 2006.

Breen G. *The Future of Management*. Boston, MA: Harvard Business School Press; 2007.

Felder C. Reality check: looking at the numbers shows where practice owners can improve. *Advance for Directors in Rehabilitation* [serial online]. 2007;16(2):13. Available at: http://rehabilitation-director.advanceweb.com/Editorial/Search/AViewer.aspx?AN=DR_07feb1_drp13.html&AD=02-01-2007. Accessed October 30, 2008.

Findly P. Plugging profitability leaks. *Advance for Directors in Rehabilitation*. 2007;16(6):19.

Glinn J. Seamless integration among all departments can maximize productivity and profits. *Advance for Directors in Rehabilitation*. 2007;17(3):14.

Keller J. Lassoing time: to make the most of your workday, follow these time management tips. *Advance for Directors in Rehabilitation*. 2002;11(8):11-12. Available at: http://rehabilitation-director.advanceweb.com/Editorial/Search/AViewer.aspx?AN=DR_02aug1_drp11.html&AD=08-01-2002. Accessed October 30, 2008.

Liebler J, McConnell C. *Management Principles for Health Professionals*. 4th Ed. Sudbury, MA: Jones and Bartlett Publishers; 2004.

Martin P, Lloyd P. Financial and operating growth strategies can solidify your practice. *Advance for Directors in Rehabilitation*. 2003;12(2):13-14.

Pozgar G. *Legal Aspects of Health Care Administration*. 10th ed. Sudbury, MA: Jones and Bartlett Publishers; 2007.

Ralls E. Get the most bang for your buck. *Online Rehab Management Journal* [serial online]. June/July 2001. Available at: http://www.rehabpub.com/features/672001/4.asp. Accessed December 8, 2008.

Scott R. *Legal Aspects of Documenting Patient Care*. 3rd ed. Sudbury, MA: Jones and Bartlett Publishers, Inc; 2006.

Winiecki B. Differential diagnosis: are you confident analyzing and dissecting the financial stability of your practice? *Advance for Directors in Rehabilitation* [serial online]. 2007;16(8):17. Available at: http://rehabilitation-director.advanceweb.com/Editorial/Search/AViewer.aspx?AN=DR_07aug1_drp17.html&AD=08-01-2007. Accessed October 30, 2008.

ELECTRONIC RESOURCES

www.inc.com: Online journal of business resources, news and emerging changes to small business.

www.redherring.com: Online in-depth analysis of economic changes, innovations, technologies, and finances.

www.sba.gov: Small business administration web portal.

CLOSING

To be successful, you must:

- Have the vision to look beyond the obvious and see the possibilities of fulfilling dreams that change the world around you, including you!

- Commit yourself to higher standards of practice, and continuously educate yourself and strive for integrity.

- Continuously improve communications with your clients, your referral sources, your employees, and your community so you can meet their expectations.

- Reduce your risk for possible litigation from clients and employees wherever possible.

- Commit to good, solid business and financial practices, and manage your money!

- Identify opportunities and emerging trends that will allow you to grow and expand your business into prevention, wellness, education, and other specialty programs that reflect the constant changing global marketplace.

WISHING YOU MUCH SUCCESS!

BUSINESS PLAN

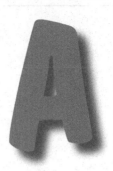

Cover Page

Business Plan

for

_____
(Name of Business)

_____
(Name of Owners)

_____
_____
_____
(Addresses and phone numbers)

_____
(Date)

_____
(Prepared by)

This plan contains information that is proprietary and confidential to _____. This obligation of confidentiality shall apply until such time that _____ make(s) the information contained in this business plan available to the public.

Business Plan Booklet © Ultimate Rehab, LLC 2001

Executive Summary

The Company

_____
_____
_____
_____
_____

The Concept

_____
_____
_____
_____
_____
_____

Products and Services

_____
_____
_____
_____
_____
_____
_____

The Market

_____
_____
_____
_____
_____

Target Market

_____
_____
_____
_____
_____
_____

(continued)

The Competition

_____
_____
_____
_____
_____
_____
_____

Management

_____
_____
_____
_____
_____
_____
_____
_____

Operations (Company's Legal Structure, Organizational Type, Practice Specialty)

_____
_____
_____
_____
_____
_____
_____
_____

Financials and Funds Sought

_____
_____
_____
_____
_____
_____
_____
_____
_____

Business Description

The Business

_____
_____
_____
_____
_____

The Business Mission

_____
_____
_____
_____
_____

Products and Services

_____
_____
_____
_____
_____

Development to Date

_____
_____
_____
_____
_____

Legal Status and Ownership

_____
_____
_____
_____

Financial Status

_____
_____
_____
_____
_____

Industry Description and Trends

Industry Analysis (External and Internal Factors)

_____
_____
_____
_____
_____
_____
_____
_____
_____
_____
_____
_____
_____

Threats to Industry

_____
_____
_____
_____
_____
_____
_____
_____

Opportunities

_____
_____
_____
_____
_____
_____
_____

Strengths (of Company in Relationship to Industry Analysis)

_____
_____
_____
_____
_____
_____
_____
_____

Target Market

Market Description
_____
_____
_____
_____
_____
_____

Market Size and Trends
_____
_____
_____
_____
_____
_____

Primary Target
_____
_____
_____
_____
_____

Secondary Target
_____
_____
_____
_____
_____

Market Readiness
_____
_____
_____
_____
_____

Opportunities
_____
_____
_____
_____
_____

Competition

Overall Description of Competitors

_____
_____
_____
_____
_____

Primary Competition

_____
_____
_____
_____
_____

Secondary Competition

_____
_____
_____
_____
_____

Advantages Over Competition

_____
_____
_____
_____
_____

Risks and Obstacles

_____
_____
_____
_____

Opportunity (in Comparison to Competitors)

_____
_____
_____
_____
_____

Marketing Plan and Strategies

Market Analysis Overall (Industry Description and Trends, Products and Services, Target Markets)

_____
_____
_____
_____
_____
_____
_____
_____
_____
_____
_____

Marketing Goals (1 to 3 years)

_____
_____
_____
_____

Marketing Strategies

_____
_____
_____
_____
_____
_____
_____
_____
_____
_____

Marketing Personnel

_____
_____
_____
_____

Management

Key Members

_____
_____
_____
_____
_____
_____
_____
_____

Staffing

_____
_____
_____
_____
_____
_____
_____
_____
_____

Consultants (Legal Counsel and Accountant)

_____
_____
_____
_____
_____
_____
_____
_____

Other Ancillary Staff (Independent Contractors, etc)

_____
_____
_____
_____
_____
_____
_____
_____
_____

Financials

List of Financial Statements

_____

_____

_____

_____

_____

_____

_____

_____

_____

_____

Attach Financial Statements to Appendix

Appendix

Supporting Documents

HOW TO START A PRIVATE PRACTICE: BREAK-EVEN ANALYSIS AND POTENTIAL MANAGEMENT ACTIONS

B

Operating Expenses (Monthly)

	Sample	Your Estimate		Source of Data	Type of Expense	Sample Assumptions
Clinical Salaries	$5,000	$5,000	You Complete	Contracted	Fixed	Single Clinician at $60K
Staff Salaries	$2,500	$2,500	You Complete	Contracted	Fixed	Single FDC at $30K
Benefits	$1,500	$1,500	Calculated	Estimated	Fixed	20% of Salaries
Clinical Supplies	$500	$500	You Complete	Estimated	Variable	
Rent	$2,000	$1,200	Calculated	Contracted	Fixed	2000 sq ft @$12
Utilities	$500	$500	You Complete	Estimated	Marginally Varia	Electric, Gas, Water
Advertising and Marketing	$500	$500	You Complete	Estimated	Variable	
Postage and Delivery	$100	$100	You Complete	Estimated	Marginally Variable	
Professional Fees	$500	$500	You Complete	Contracted	Variable	
Telephone	$150	$150	You Complete	Estimated	Marginally Variable	
Laundry and Cleaning	$120	$120	You Complete	Estimated	Marginally Variable	
Maintenance and Repairs	$250	$250	You Complete	Estimated	Marginally Variable	
Insurance	$180	$180	You Complete	Contracted	Fixed	
Depreciation	$600	$600	You Complete	Contracted	Fixed	Start up Expenses
Principal and Interest Expense	$2,500	$2,500	You Complete	Contracted	Fixed	13.4% of Salaries
FICA	$1,005	$1,005	Calculated	Contracted	Fixed	
Misc	$500	$500	You Complete	Estimated	Variable	
Total	$18,405	$17,605				

Size of Clinic $1,200
Lease Rate $12

Break Even Calculations

	Typical	Improved Collections	Improved Write Offs	Improved Collections and Write Offs	Best Practice	Your Estimates	Sample Assumptions
Gross Charge per Visit	$100	$100	$100	$100	$125	$100	You Complete
Bad Debt Write Off	25%	25%	15%	15%	10%	25%	You Complete
Collection Rate	65%	75%	65%	75%	90%	65%	You Complete
Average Charge per Visit	$100	$100	$100	$100	$125	$100	Calculated
Estimated Write-off	$25	$25	$15	$15	$13	$25	Calculated
Net Charge per Visit	$75	$75	$85	$85	$113	$75	Calculated
Est. Reimb per Visit	$49	$56	$55	$64	$101	$49	Calculated

Operating Income

	Typical	Improved Collections	Improved Write Offs	Improved Collections and Write Offs	Best Practice	Your Estimates	Sample Assumptions
Net Operating Income	$18,405	$18,405	$18,405	$18,405	$18,405	$17,605	Calculated
Billing and Collection Cost Rate	20%	25%	25%	30%	15%	20%	You Complete
Billing and Collection Costs	$3,681	$4,601	$4,601	$5,522	$2,761	$3,521	Calculated
Required Revenue	$22,086	$23,006	$23,006	$23,927	$21,166	$21,126	Calculated

Breakeven Analysis

	Typical	Improved Collections	Improved Write Offs	Improved Collections and Write Offs	Best Practice	Your Estimates	Sample Assumptions
Required Revenue	$22,086	$23,006	$23,006	$23,927	$21,166	$21,126	Calculated
Reimbursement per Visit	$49	$56	$55	$64	$101	$49	Calculated
Required Visits per Month	453.0	409.0	416.4	375.3	209.0	433.4	Calculated
Visits per day to B/E (21.5days/mo)	21.1	19.0	19.4	17.5	9.7	20.2	Calculated

Potential Management Actions

	Impact	Impact Apparent
1. Enhance Clinician Product	High	Future Payroll
2. Lower Supply Expenses	Low	Supplies
3. Improve Payer Mix	High	Collection Rate and Write Off
4. Adjust Salaries	Medium	Payroll
5. Increase Collectibles	High	Collection Rate
6. Lower Costs of Collection	Medium	Billing and Collection Costs

SAMPLES OF MARKETING MATERIALS

C

**CAMARILLO AQUATIC AND
REHABILITATION SERVICES**

Dave Powers MA MBA PT
Director and Owner

1583 Calle Patricia Ste 200   Tel: 888-REHAB-53
Pacific Palisades, CA 90272   Fax: 310-454-5049

Business card

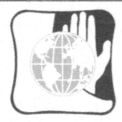

ABC WELLNESS
Paradise, USA
800-GET-WELL

GIFT CERTIFICATE

This certificate entitles CLIENT   *to* 1 MASSAGE

Authorized by

Expires Happy Mother's Day!!

Gift certificate

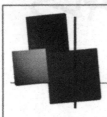

ORTHOPEDICS
INTERNATIONAL INC.

9735 Wilshire Blvd. Ste 421
Beverly Hills, CA 90212
Tel: 310.275.8480
Fax: 310.274.1815

Business magnet

Advertisement Heading

Use this space to tell your readers about your business, product, service, or event. This text should tell the reader what your offer can do for them.	**List your featured Items** • list item here • list item here • list item here • list item here

ABC REHAB

List your hours or the time and date of your event. Describe your location by landmark or area of town.

Tel: 555 555 5555

Newspaper ad

THANK YOU

October 15, 2001

Ultimate Rehab would like to thank all of you who stopped by our booth in Sacramento . It was exciting to meet everyone and hear about your interests in private practice.

We invite you to email us with your questions and feedback on how we may better serve your small business, private practice needs. Our goal is to make our company, *www.ultimaterehab.com*, your one stop, rehab source for health and business solutions.

Check out this month's article on : **"Documentation Compliance; Where Do I Start?"**

Our **Feature Product** this month is the **LIFEPAK 500 AED;** Workplace Safety Program. Special pricing/leasing available.

Motivation Tip #1: Step into new opportunities with an open mind for unthinkable possibilities!

We look forward to hearing you!

Tammy Richmond MS OTR and Dave Powers MBA MA PT
www.ultimaterehab.com
Ultimate Rehab, LLC
888-REHAB-53
info@ultimaterehab.com

Postcard (email or postal)

IMPLEMENTATION TOOLS

Leasing Worksheet

Leasing a location requires attention to details. It is important to read the lease agreement very carefully. In most cases, you should have your attorney review the lease with you. Be sure that you fully understand all aspects of the lease. The following is a list of points you need to consider when leasing:

- What are the terms of the lease?
- What is the cost per square foot per month?
- Does it include all expenses (triple net versus gross lease versus percentage lease)?
- How long is the lease?
- Do you have the option to renew the lease?
- Do you have the option to sublease to others?
- What is the condition of the premises (eg, does it have utilities and are they in working condition)?
- Who will pay for tenant improvements (should these be negotiated)?
- Is parking or parking validation included in the cost of the lease?
- What is your ability to access the premises (24 hours a day, 7 days a week, 52 weeks per year)?
- Are you allowed to put up signage? If yes, what are the restrictions?
- When do you have to start paying for the space? (It is important to determine how long it will take to complete the building of your new clinic. Try to negotiate payments starting sometime after the project is completed and you have started to bring in revenue.)

Once you have signed the lease, it is important to find a contractor who can oversee the building of the clinic. The contractor should be very experienced with building small businesses, preferably health care practices.

The following steps are important as you proceed with your project:

- ❏ Interview contractors.
- ❏ Check references.
- ❏ Look at projects they have completed.
- ❏ Discuss a price and payment plan.
- ❏ Secure a written contract that includes time lines for the completion of the clinic. (It is important to have your attorney review the contract prior to signing.)
- ❏ When paying for subcontractors, make sure your checks are written to the contractor and the subcontractor. (This prevents the contractor from not paying the subcontractors and leaving you responsible for a second payment.)
- ❏ Do not make your final payment to your contractor until your project is 100% complete.

Liability Insurance Information

Obtain professional liability insurance:

- The Healthcare Provider's Service Organization at 888-288-3534 (endorsed by the APTA)
- Seabury and Smith (Marsh Affinity) 800-503-9230 (endorsed by the AOTA)

  [NOTE: Both insurance companies may be available for both professions; varies by state.]

Applying for coverage:

- Talk with other therapists about carriers they are using. Have they had any situations where they had to engage with the insurance company?
- Speak to representatives from all insurance companies about your particular needs.
- Obtain the appropriate forms and information.
- Carefully read the policy information and understand all of the inclusions and exclusions.
- Be sure to find out what notice provisions are required.
- Fill out the application completely, even if it means including embarrassing information.
- Don't leave questions blank; use N/A.
- Talk with the insurance agent if you have questions while completing the application.
- Once you receive the copy of proof, make copies and store them in a safe and accessible place.

Adequate coverage:
- Discuss and understand your policy with your insurer.
- Assess your practice for any activities you perform that aren't covered.
- Purchase "tail coverage" for extended periods to report claims (claims-made).
- Purchase additional coverage to cover "other" activities.

Questions to ask your employer and/or insurer:
- Am I covered by a claims-made or by an occurrence policy (ie, if my employer were to change policies, would a later claim for an incident that occurred during the previous policy's term be covered by that previous policy)? If my coverage is a claims-made policy, are there any gaps in my coverage?
- What is your definition of a "claim"?
- If I were named as a defendant in a lawsuit (against my employer), would I be assigned my own attorney?
- What are the limits of liability for each incident?
- How many other professional employees or support employees share in the limits of liability?
- What are the aggregate limits of liability each year for the practice setting?
- What are the areas of exclusion?
- If I terminate my employment, will the coverage provided by my former employer's policy protect me from claims resulting from an incident when I was employed?
- If my employer merges with another employer, what assurances do I have that I will be covered for incidents prior to the merger?
- What happens to my insurance if my employer (or I) closes the practice or goes bankrupt?
- What happens to my insurance protection if my employer (or I) fails to pay the insurance premium on the employer policy?
- Will my employer's (or my) policy cover me for physical therapy practices other than at my place of employment?
- Will I be covered for acts construed to be outside the scope of my employment?
- Will I be supported by the employer's policy only if the employer supports my conduct at the time of the incident?
- Do I have personal injury protection for acts of libel, slander, or defamation?
- Do I have personal liability protection for acts that can be construed as nonprofessional?
- Will I be covered for legal representation if I am brought before my state licensing board for a disciplinary hearing as a result of a professional liability incident?

Updating your coverage:
- File your policy in a safe but accessible place.
- Make sure to pay your premium on time.
- Evaluate your practice and policy annually.
- If moving, check to make sure your present policy complies with the new state location.

Obtain other necessary insurance:
- General liability; errors/omissions
- Business owner's packages
- Equipment insurance
- Workers' compensation
- Commercial auto insurance
- Employment practice coverage

BUYING OR SELLING A PRACTICE

Items to be reviewed:

- Federal Income Tax Returns (last 3 years)

- Financial Statements (current balance statement, monthly operating costs sheet, income statement)

- Number of Treatment Procedures (per day, per month, per year)

- Gross Per Month (last two years)

- Number of Clients per month (last two years)

- Number of New Clients per month (last two years)

- Number of Referring Physicians (last two years)

- Staffing (type, wage, benefits given)

- Production Per Therapist per month (last two years)

- Current Payroll Journal (include position & hire date)

- Fee Schedule (copy of fee schedule for each insurance carrier per contract)

- List of Major Medical Equipment

- List of Office Equipment

- Appraisal of Equipment (resale value)

- Appraisal of Building or Space, if owned

- Lease (how long, how much, when to be renewed)

- Estimation of Supplies on Hand (amount and resale value)

REHAB BUSINESS EQUIPMENT LIST

Hydro
- Aquatic rehab equipment
- Whirlpools
- Underwater treadmills
- Pools-prefab

Modalities
- Diathermy
- Ultrasound
- Phoresor/iontophoresis
- Interferential unit
- Muscle stimulator
- TENS/FES
- Paraffin bath/wax
- Biofeedback
- Hot/cold packs

Treatment Equipment
- Wall pulleys
- Stair climbers
- Treadmills
- Bikes
- Upper cycles
- Floor mats
- Free weights
- Parallel bars
- Weight stations
- Traction units
- Mat tables
- Step stools
- Total gym

Treatment Tables
- Electric hi-lo table
- Wooden plinths
- Tilt tables
- Mat tables
- OT work tables
- Massage table

Miscellaneous Equipment
- Cabinetry
- Charts/models
- Mobile carts
- Weight scale
- Dynamometer
- Pinch meter
- Reflex hammer
- Blood pressure and stethoscope
- Exam stools
- Cubicle curtains
- Office furniture
- Lobby furniture
- Art work for the walls
- Staff room table and chairs
- Refrigerator
- Microwave
- Fax machine
- Copier
- Computers
- Phone system

Miscellaneous Supplies
- Office supplies
- Timers
- Call bells
- Tape measure
- Patient gowns
- Towels
- Pillows
- Positioning wedges

FACILITY CHECKLIST

❏   Reception room

❏   Business office (allow for fax, computer, copier, and plenty of storage)

❏   Manager's office

❏   Waiting room

❏   Confidential storage of medical records

❏   Linen storage (clean and dirty)

❏   Washer and dryer (you may want to send out your dirty linen)

❏   Restrooms (patient and staff)

❏   Gym (determine equipment needed and how it will fit into your space)
   • Consider mirrors
   • Need sink and drinking water

❏   Treatment rooms (curtains versus solid walled) (remember HIPAA and the importance of private evaluations)
   • Size at least 10' x 10'
   • Built-in cabinets versus moveable ones

❏   Sound system
   • Intercom/page system
   • Music system

❏   Emergency call system

❏   Hydro (keep near your restrooms to decrease plumbing cost)
   • Individual tanks
   • Pool
   • Review federal, state, and local codes for pool installation
   • Determine if you have the option to heat with electric or gas (gas is cheaper in most cases)
   • Needs floor drainage

❏   Work room (include hot/cold pack machine, refrigerator/ice machine)

❏   Housekeeping room (store equipment and supplies to clean the clinic)

❏   Storage room (this is an area that is often overlooked)
   • Crutches
   • Walkers
   • Canes
   • Electrical stimulator
   • Ultrasound
   • Tens
   • Phoresor
   • Other durable medical equipment
   • Office supplies
   • Cleaning supplies
   • TV/VCR/DVD player

❏   Staff room (most staff should have their own area for storing personal items and doing their documentation)

❏   Break room (consider refrigerator, microwave, and an area for staff to eat)

❏   Conference room

❏   Electrical (it is important to put as many plugs as you think you may need during construction; they become very expensive to add after the project is complete)
   • Four plugs in each treatment room—36" high
   • Plugs every 6' in gym—36" high

❑ Computer network (consider all areas where you think you may want a computer because it is much less expensive to wire the clinic for computers during construction than after it is completed)
- Manager's office
- Business office
- Staff room
- Gym
- Conference room

❑ Lighting
- Individual lighting controls in all treatment rooms with dimmer switches

❑ Phone system (may also be used for your intercom system)
- Business office
- Gym
- Break room
- Waiting room

❑ Security system

❑ Signage
- Check with local laws, making sure your signage meets the codes

POLICY AND PROCEDURE MANUAL: GENERAL POLICIES

- Mission statement
- Vision statement
- Sexual harassment
- Progressive disciplinary action
- Employee orientation
- Informed consent
- Documentation
- Unusual occurrence report
- Discharge from therapy
- HIPAA privacy regulations
- Compliance plan
- Work rules
- Dress code
- Hours of operation
- Staff development
- Employee payroll
- Vacation, sick, and holiday time
- Employee injury
- Job descriptions
- Performance evaluations
- Personnel files
- Competency evaluations
- Professional liability insurance
- Telephone usage/Internet usage/radio usage/television usage
- Standards of care
- Referral
- Treatment frequency and duration
- Quality assurance plan
- Peer review
- Home program
- Use of equipment
- Infection control/safety procedures
- Fire safety procedure/disaster plan
- Medical emergency response
- Patients rights and responsibilities
- Release of medical information
- Cancellation policy
- Treatment protocols
- Billing
- Reimbursement

INFORMED CONSENT

Orthopedic and Sports Physical Therapy

Physical therapy is a patient care service provided in response to a wide range of medical care needs of outpatients of all ages, regardless of gender, color, ethnicity, creed, national origin, or disability.

The purpose of physical therapy is to treat disease, injury, and disability by examination, evaluation, diagnosis, prognosis, and intervention by use of rehabilitative procedures, by mobilization, massage, exercises, and physical agents to aid the patient in achieving their maximum potential within their capabilities, and to accelerate convalescence and reduce the length of the functional recovery. All procedures will be thoroughly explained to you before you are asked to perform them.

You are expected to cooperate fully with the evaluation and treatment program. Because of the nature of services provided, you might be asked to disrobe. If this is necessary, your privacy, modesty, and dignity will be considered at all times by the staff. Should you feel uncomfortable or embarrassed, you may refuse the procedure, stop the procedure, and/or request another therapist.

There are certain inherent risks with physical therapy treatments because you will be asked to exert effort and perform activities with increasing degrees of difficulty that could cause an increase in your current level of pain, discomfort, or an aggravation to your existing injury. You will be able to stop treatment if you feel any discomfort or pain. Your physical therapist will take every precaution to ensure that you are protected from any potentially hazardous situation. You will never be forced to perform any procedure that you do not wish to perform.

Based on the above information, I agree to cooperate fully, to participate in all physical therapy procedures, and to comply with the plan of care as it is established. I have read and received a copy of the consent form and authorize release of medical information to appropriate third parties.

Client's Signature_____ Date _____

UNUSUAL OCCURRENCE REPORT

Complete the following items:

Client's name _____

Location of occurrence _____

Witness_____

Person completing form_____

Date of occurrence_____

Time of occurrence _____

Description of occurrence (briefly describe what happened and the outcome):
_____
_____
_____

Manager's investigation/analysis:
_____
_____
_____

Action taken:
_____
_____
_____

This Report Is Confidential

Not A Part Of Medical Record

Do Not Photocopy

WHAT QUESTIONS SHOULD YOU ASK
WHEN CONSIDERING MEMBERSHIP IN A NETWORK?

- How long has the network been operational?
- Does the network have a Board of Directors? If so, who are they and what is their profession?
- Who owns and operates the network?
- Does the network require exclusivity?
- What is the network retention of records?
- What is the network claim submission process?
- What is the network's compliance program?
- How does the network audit and monitor its work?
- How does the network maintain the integrity of its data systems?
- What are the network's policies and procedures?
- Who is the staff, and what type of training and education do they have?
- Have there been any legal claims against the network?
- What are the annual dues, and how are they spent by the network?
- How many providers does the network represent, and in what discipline?
- Is a network representative assigned to my clinic?
- Do they have an office in my geographical area? If not, will the representative visit my clinic to discuss problems/ concerns; or, what type of communication will there be?
- What is the network's mission, and does it match my clinic's philosophy?
- What services will the network perform for my clinic?
- How many managed care contracts does the network hold, and how many does each have in my clinic's service area?
- What type of reimbursement has the network negotiated?
- Will my clinic have a choice regarding participation in managed care contracts?
- Read the network's participation contract carefully. Does the contract allow me to maintain my clinic's autonomy? Does it allow me to pursue individual managed care contracts if I leave the network?

QUESTIONS TO ASK MEDICAL BILLERS OR
MEDICAL BILLING SERVICES BEFORE CONTRACTING WITH THEM

- How long has the individual or company been operational?
- Who owns and operates the company?
- How does the company retain records? Are they secure and private?
- What is the company's HIPAA policy?
- What is the cost structure agreement (ie, what percentage does the company charge for billing services, second claims processing, etc. Ask for entire cost structure and schedule of fees)?
- What is the company's claim submission process?
- How does the company monitor and audit its work?
- Who are the staff, and what type of training and education do they have?
- Have there been legal claims against the company?
- What is the set-up cost?
- What are the percentages charged for collections?
- How many health care providers does the company presently represent?
- What disciplines do they represent?
- What type of patient populations, diagnosis, and third-party payers do they routinely bill for and to?
- How often will they communicate with me?
- How often will they bill for me?
- What is the average turnaround time for a claim?
- What do they do in case of denials?
- What additional services do they provide (ie, negotiating with third-party payers)?
- How do I begin and terminate relationships with the company (ie, contract or termination clauses)?
- Do they have a company résumé and at least three references they can send me?
- Do they have professional liability insurance or some type of insurance policy (ask for proof of insurance)?
- Ask the references they provide the following:
  o What type of patient populations are serviced and billed?
  o How many denials?
  o How does the biller communicate?
  o Do they have any concerns?

INTERVIEW QUESTIONS

Ask each applicant to provide you with a current résumé and at least three references. Call each of the references. If they have a license, certification, or credentials, be sure it is current. Ask if there have ever been any problems with their license in this state or any other state.

Consider the following as you put together your interview questions:

- What characteristics are important to you?
- What type of work setting is this applicant interested in?
    - Type of supervision
    - Type of patients
    - Type of setting… etc
- How does he or she feel about working with an assistant and/or aides?
- What are his or her professional goals?
- What are his or her strengths?
- What are his or her weaknesses?
- How does he or she feel about working in a start-up company?
- Ask about his or her internships.
- How does he or she deal with doctor or therapist conflicts?
- How does he or she deal with peer conflict?
- How does he or she deal with constructive feedback?
- How does he or she feel about working and/or treating people with diverse backgrounds?
- Is he or she comfortable with starting off with a per diem or independent status?
- What does he or she expect as an hourly wage?

It is important that you have a relaxed atmosphere for the interview. Be honest with the applicant. Describe the organization and your expectations for the position. If you paint a picture that is different than what your clinic really presents, the employee will not last. The applicant should be doing most of the talking during the interview.

If you decide to hire the applicant, extend an offer in writing. Be willing to be flexible in your offer, but be fair to other individuals already on staff. Put everything you agree upon in writing and have the new hire sign the agreement. A copy should be given to the employee and a copy kept in his or her employee file.

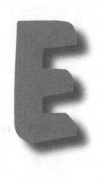

DOCUMENTATION
SELF-ASSESSMENT

Documentation
Self – Assessment

**Rate Your Practice In These Key Indicators Of Documentation Success
Now and Where You Need to Be to Succeed.**

Instructions

Score yourself on each of the following indicators listed in the first column.
Indicate the extent that your typical current practices and your future ideal practices match the indicator in the second column.
Note the difference between your actual and ideal in the third column.
In the last column, indicate how important this indicator really is in your practice.

Key Indicator	Score Actual and Ideal	Difference Actual/Ideal (Ideal–Actual)	Importance of Indicator (A, B, C)
Mechanics	"Medicare covers outpatient physical therapy, occupational therapy, and speech pathology services rendered. The guidelines state that the services must be reasonable and necessary to treat an individual's illness or injury. There must be an expectation that the patient's condition will improve significantly in a reasonable and generally predictable period of time, and the services must relate directly to the treatment goals. In addition, the services must be at a level of complexity and sophistication that they can be safely and effectively rendered only by (or under the supervision of) a skilled therapist."		
My notes are legible.	Strongly Agree Strongly Disagree 1 2 3 4 5		
My notes are completed in a timely manner.	Strongly Agree Strongly Disagree 1 2 3 4 5		
Every treatment that I perform is documented in my notes.	Strongly Agree Strongly Disagree 1 2 3 4 5		
Every supply item or piece of equipment that I provide is documented in my notes.	Strongly Agree Strongly Disagree 1 2 3 4 5		
Every treatment session has a note.	Strongly Agree Strongly Disagree 1 2 3 4 5		
My documentation is timely, legible and complete.	Strongly Agree Strongly Disagree 1 2 3 4 5		
My documentation clearly articulates the skill and medical necessity of the services I provide.	Strongly Agree Strongly Disagree 1 2 3 4 5		

Plan of Care and Goals	"Patient care that is inadequately documented will be considered patient care that was never provided. Long-term success requires ongoing diligence to clearly explain why rehabilitation therapy was required for the patient to succeed."		
	Score **Actual and Ideal**	**Ideal–Actual**	**A, B, C**
My plan of care is based on a thorough and concise evaluation.	Strongly Agree Strongly Disagree 1 2 3 4 5		
My documentation clearly articulates the skill and medical necessity of the services I provide.	Strongly Agree Strongly Disagree 1 2 3 4 5		
We have standards for documentation and systems to assure that those standards are met.	Strongly Agree Strongly Disagree 1 2 3 4 5		
My goals are objective, functional, time-based and measurable.	Strongly Agree Strongly Disagree 1 2 3 4 5		
Our documentation complies with accreditation and regulatory agency requirements.	Strongly Agree Strongly Disagree 1 2 3 4 5		
When necessary, our documentation provides a solid base upon which to form an appeal.	Strongly Agree Strongly Disagree 1 2 3 4 5		

Medical Necessity	"Medicare pays for outpatient physical therapy, occupational therapy, and speech pathology services that are reasonable and necessary for the treatment of an individual's illness or injury"		
I am careful to document why the patient requires my care.	Strongly Agree Strongly Disagree 1 2 3 4 5		
My documentation clearly states the patient's potential for improvement.	Strongly Agree Strongly Disagree 1 2 3 4 5		
My documentation estimates the amount of improvement that is anticipated in functional terms.	Strongly Agree Strongly Disagree 1 2 3 4 5		

Skill Level	"Medicare requires the provider to demonstrate that the services were: (1) medically reasonable and necessary for the patient to improve; (2) furnished under a treatment plan that has been reviewed by a physician; (3) furnished while the patient was under the continuous care of a physician; (4) be of such intensity and complexity that the skills of a qualified therapist are required."		
	Score Actual and Ideal	**Ideal–Actual**	**A, B, C**
My documentation demonstrates that the care I provide requires the skills of a therapist.	Strongly Agree 1 2 3 Strongly Disagree 4 5		
I actively participate in efforts to improve our documentation practices.	Strongly Agree 1 2 3 Strongly Disagree 4 5		
I am confident that our bills to payers match the documentation that I provide.	Strongly Agree 1 2 3 Strongly Disagree 4 5		

Coding Practices	"Coding the care appropriately is the obvious next step in describing your services in a manner that is likely to be reimbursed. Describe your care inappropriately and it is likely that you will not be reimbursed correctly."		
In all cases my notes and billing match.	Strongly Agree 1 2 3 Strongly Disagree 4 5		
I have current knowledge of coding practices.	Strongly Agree 1 2 3 Strongly Disagree 4 5		
I understand the coding requirements of different payers.	Strongly Agree 1 2 3 Strongly Disagree 4 5		
My organization routinely verifies that our coding practice is current and appropriate.	Strongly Agree 1 2 3 Strongly Disagree 4 5		
We have systems to train staff about appropriate coding practices.	Strongly Agree 1 2 3 Strongly Disagree 4 5		

Action Planning

Which areas are most problematic for you based on the difference between your actual performance and what you identified as ideal?

_____
_____
_____
_____
_____
_____
_____
_____
_____

Which of those did you rate as the most important?

_____
_____
_____
_____
_____

What actions will you take to address the areas that you've identified as both problematic and important?

_____
_____
_____
_____
_____

What support systems will need to be in place to help you succeed as you address your problem areas?

_____
_____
_____
_____
_____
_____
_____
_____
_____

PRODUCTIVITY SELF-ASSESSMENT

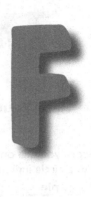

The Productivity Quiz

Rate Yourself as The Productive Therapist - Now and Where You Plan to Be.

Score yourself on each of the following characteristics.
Put a circle indicating where you are now and an X where you want to be.

Example	Never	Sometimes		Always
I am as productive as I can be without lowering the quality of my patient care.	1_____2_____	3 _____	_4_____	5

Handling Interruptions Throughout My Day	Never	Sometimes		Always
I have systems to limit interruptions throughout my day	1_____2_____	3_____	4_____	5
I notify the office which situations or calls warrant interruptions	1_____2_____	3_____	4_____	5
I schedule specific times to return calls	1_____2_____	3_____	4_____	5
I schedule specific times to receive calls	1_____2_____	3_____	4_____	5
I share clinical techniques only for professional reasons - never for social reasons	1_____2_____	3_____	4_____	5
I am able to focus on my clinical care. I am not easily distracted in the clinic	1_____2_____	3_____	4_____	5

Scheduling and Organizing My Day	Never	Sometimes		Always
I schedule my patients in regular time slots when possible	1_____2_____	3_____	4_____	5
I am aware of my schedule for the day	1_____2_____	3_____	4_____	5
I anticipate discharges and plan accordingly	1_____2_____	3_____	4_____	5
I have a system to prioritize my tasks, such as a daily planner	1_____2_____	3_____	4_____	5
I prepare at the end of each day for the next day's activities	1_____2_____	3_____	4_____	5
I prepare at the end of each morning for my afternoon activities	1_____2_____	3_____	4_____	5

Reproduced with permission of Kovacek Management Services. www.ptmanager.com.

Structuring My Initial Patient Interactions

	Never		Sometimes		Always
I explain the importance of attendance to each patient at the time of the initial evaluation	1	2	3	4	5
I do not give patients "permission" to cancel appointments or fail to show	1	2	3	4	5
I help my patients develop a mental picture of what success in therapy will be for them	1	2	3	4	5
I work with my patients as a partner to them to develop mutual goals	1	2	3	4	5
I negotiate agreement and commitment to our mutual goals with my patients	1	2	3	4	5
I emphasize patient responsibility and the need for a team effort for optimal recovery	1	2	3	4	5

Structuring My Ongoing Patient Interactions

	Never		Sometimes		Always
I am committed to patient education	1	2	3	4	5
I use educational handouts, demonstrations, and audiovisuals to make my patient teaching more effective	1	2	3	4	5
I personalize handouts for each patient by highlighting those areas most important for that patient	1	2	3	4	5
I back up verbal instruction with written materials	1	2	3	4	5
I determine my patient's commitment to completion of home programs and to following recommendations	1	2	3	4	5
I ask my patients about their actual success in performing home programs and following recommendations	1	2	3	4	5
I use simple language and avoid jargon and multi syllable words in my explanations to my patients	1	2	3	4	5
I remind myself to listen more and talk less with my patients	1	2	3	4	5
I work to improve my listening skills, including maintaining good eye contact with my patients	1	2	3	4	5

My Treatment Philosophy

	Never		Sometimes		Always
I emphasize what works rather than any specific set of clinical techniques	1	2	3	4	5
I emphasize the patient's role in their recovery	1	2	3	4	5
I define quality from the patient's perspective, not mine	1	2	3	4	5
I define good therapy as what produces the best and quickest results	1	2	3	4	5
I use a tiered approach to patient care, starting with the least costly, least risky treatments when I am unsure of a single, best course of action	1	2	3	4	5

Meetings

	Never		Sometimes		Always
I attend meetings on time	1	2	3	4	5
I request timed agendas for meetings that I attend	1	2	3	4	5
I participate in meeting effectiveness critiques to improve our meeting processes	1	2	3	4	5

My Documentation

	Never		Sometimes		Always
I complete my notes while I am with the patients	1	2	3	4	5
I use documentation technology to my benefit, not to my detriment	1	2	3	4	5
I keep up with my notes, I rarely fall significantly behind	1	2	3	4	5

My Delegation Style

	Never		Sometimes		Always
I delegate routine or repetitive care	1	2	3	4	5
I communicate with support staff to receive feedback on the patient's response to treatment	1	2	3	4	5
I use a decision process to decide what, when and to whom to delegate	1	2	3	4	5

The Productivity Quiz

Planning Sheet

Section	Who Will Help	Actions Needed to Improve	Time Frame
Handling Interruptions			
Scheduling and Organizing			
Initial Patient Interactions			
Ongoing Patient Interactions			
Treatment Philosophy			
Meetings			
Documentation			
Delegation Style			

If there is a difference between where you think you are now and where you want to be, you need to change some of your activities and/or attitudes to reach what you have identified as where you want to be. These are your targets, no one else's.

Developing a plan to bridge the gap in where you are and where you want to be.

What actions will you take to change your behaviors and skills as a productive clinician? List them here.

_____
_____
_____

When do you want to accomplish this? Be specific.

_____
_____
_____

Who will help and support you as you make these changes?

_____
_____
_____

Good Luck as you become The Productive Therapist.

MANAGEMENT AND OPERATIONS CHECKLIST

G

Management and Operations Checklist

- ❐ Professional licenses and certifications renewals in personnel file
- ❐ Professional PDUs/CEUs completed and in personnel file
- ❐ Professional liability insurance for each therapist, practice
- ❐ General commercial insurance
- ❐ Workers' compensation insurance
- ❐ Business license renewal
- ❐ Yearly property taxes
- ❐ Quarterly federal tax return
- ❐ Quarterly contribution return (EDD)
- ❐ Quarterly wage and withholding report
- ❐ Secretary of State; Corporation fee
- ❐ Yearly corporation federal and state tax return
- ❐ Business checking account in name of business
- ❐ Accounting software for invoicing or billing
- ❐ Independent contractor agreements (if applicable)
- ❐ Job descriptions
- ❐ Business description
- ❐ Documentation requirements (Code of Ethics, Standards of Practice, Copy of Laws and Regulations, Practice Guidelines, Intake Form, Consent to Treatment, HIPAA Privacy Form, Patient Rights Form, Cancellation Policy, Notice to Payment)
- ❐ Obtain Medicare or other government-funded application and approval PTAN number for practice and each therapist (855I); Reassignment of individual therapists PTAN to practice (855R); Change in ownership/management (855I); Deactivation of PTANs (855R)
- ❐ DMERC contract and numbers (PTAN, NPI)
- ❐ EFT contract and procedures updated
- ❐ NPI numbers for practice, each therapist, and DME
- ❐ Contracts with third party payers current and on file
- ❐ Labor law review; overtime log, time alteration log, patient sign in log, time off log, holiday and benefit log, PTO log.
- ❐ Part-time or full-time benefits current policy and documentation
- ❐ Policy and procedure manual
- ❐ OSHA and universal safety policy and manual, and postings
- ❐ Chart review
- ❐ Outcome measurements
- ❐ Patient satisfaction surveys
- ❐ Equipment calibration service log
- ❐ Equipment and modalities maintenance log
- ❐ Emergency procedures
- ❐ Medical record and safety tracking procedures
- ❐ Employee contracts
- ❐ Billing
  - ○ Prescription or referral, if indicated
  - ○ Superbill
  - ○ Supply sheets/costs
  - ○ Evaluation/assessment documentation

(continued)

- o Daily encounter note (Time in/time out)
- o 30-day progress note
- o Discharge summary
- o Denial, restriction, and delay procedures
- o Scope of practice/Evidence-based support materials
- o Code restrictions noted
- o EOB posting procedures
- o Aging accounts procedures
- o Billing and coding changes retrieval procedures
- o Recertification/re-credentialing of therapists w/payers

❑ Accounting
- o Income/expense daily, monthly
- o Budget
- o Payroll (see above reports required)
- o Independent contractors or per diem accounting
- o Shareholder accounting

❑ Human Resources
- o Hiring/firing procedures
- o Peer review
- o Wage increase
- o Benefits qualification
- o Employee handbook
- o Disciplinary actions/procedures
- o Staffing development/Staff meetings

❑ Marketing
- o Marketing strategies (business cards, brochures, ads, website, etc)
- o Marketing budget
- o Marketing tasks procedures (who, when, how often)

SOLE PROPRIETORSHIP START-UP

SOLE PROPRIETORSHIP (ONE OWNER, NO EMPLOYEES)

Steps to Start-Up

- ☐ Obtain professional licenses and certifications
- ☐ Professional liability insurance
- ☐ DBA for business
- ☐ Business license in the city district of business address
- ☐ Business checking account in name of business
- ☐ Accounting software for invoicing or billing
- ☐ Independent contractor agreement (if applicable)
- ☐ Job description
- ☐ Business description
- ☐ Documentation requirements (code of ethics, standards of practice, copy of laws and regulations, practice guidelines, etc)
- ☐ Obtain Medicare or other government-funded application and approval PIN
- ☐ Contracts with third-party payers (if applicable)
- ☐ Work calendar
- ☐ Mileage log
- ☐ Expense log
- ☐ File quarterly and annual taxes

ELECTRONIC RESOURCES

Business Fundamentals for the Rehabilitation Professional, Second Edition answers the "what, where, how, and when" questions of transforming a health care practice idea into a successful business. Designed to integrate small business guidelines with health care regulations, practice operations, and management, this text is perfect for rehabilitation professionals and entrepreneurs interested in starting up or expanding their practice businesses. To help update the book, the authors have provided pertinent web addresses to give the reader access to the most current information possible about each topic listed in the book

PLEASE VISIT
HTTP://www.routledge.com/9781556428838/BUSINESSFUNDAMENTALS

GLOSSARY

abilities: Qualities that are inherent, learned, accomplished, and needed.

accounts payable: Accounts of businesses representing obligations to pay for goods and services received.

accounts receivable: Accounts of businesses representing moneys due for goods sold or services rendered, evidenced by notes, statements, invoices, or other written evidence of a present obligation.

accrual basis: The more popular method of accounting in which income or expenses are recorded at the time they occur, not when they are received.

advertising: Any paid form of written promotion for your products or services.

angel: A private individual who invests his or her own money in new enterprises.

assets: Those resources and experiences that can be used to your advantage. Documentation of property leased or purchased for your business to verify annual depreciation, costs, or sales expenses.

break-even analysis: The evaluation of the relationship between costs, volume, and profits.

business plan: A comprehensive planning document that clearly describes the business developmental objective of an existing or proposed business.

business structure: The organizational outcome of several business tasks that legally defines a business entity.

capital: The funds necessary to establish or operate a business.

cash basis: A method of accounting in which income is counted when the payment is actually received, not when you bill it or invoice it.

cash flow: The movement of money into and out of a company; actual income received and actual payments made out.

code of ethics: Public statement of the common set of values and principles used to promote and maintain high standards of behavior in occupational and physical therapy.

corporation: A group of persons granted a state charter, legally recognizing it as a separate entity having its own rights, privileges, and liabilities distinct from those of its members. The process of incorporating should be completed with the state's secretary of state or state corporate counsel and usually requires the services of an attorney.

debt financing: Raising funds for a business by borrowing, often in the form of bank loans.

desires: Something you would pursue if you knew how to do so, or your personal interests you want to pursue.

domain name: Synonymous with the term "Web site name."

employment tax: Federal income tax withholding, social security and medicare taxes (FICA), and federal unemployment (FUTA) tax.

entrepreneur: One who assumes the financial risk of the initiation, operation, and management of a given business or undertaking.

equity: An ownership interest in a business.

exit plan: The strategy for leaving an investment and realizing the profits of such investment.

expenses: Documents that show the costs to operate a business, such as receipts, account statements, invoices, and tax records.

explanation of benefits (EOB): Statement of policy holder's health care benefits regarding health care services received and paid.

federal employee identification number (EIN): Taxpayer identification number that is assigned by the IRS. It is required under certain business circumstances.

fictitious business name (Doing Business As [DBA]): The name under which you will be conducting business.

financial reports: Reports commonly required from applicants for financial assistance, such as balance sheets, income statement, and cash flow.

fixed expenses (costs): Costs that do not vary from month to month based on usage, often referred to as "overhead costs."

for-profit: Providing services and products for the purpose of making money for owners.

gross receipts: Those income receipts that you receive from your business, such as invoices, cash and credit card receipts, bank deposit slips, and check stubs.

HIPAA notice of privacy policy: A statement given to patients to inform them of their privacy rights with respect to their personal health information. The notice must also be visibly posted in the practice.

income tax: Tax paid on monies or profits made.

informed consent: This form explains the treatment process and provides an avenue of communication to assist in risk management.

legal corporate and company name: The name you choose to incorporate and register with the Secretary of State.

legal structure: The organizational formations of specific legal business tasks and documentation that define elements of ownership or the relationship between owners, types of businesses and business objectives, management, and legal operations.

licensing or certification laws and regulations: Sets of rules and policies that govern rehab professionals established at the state government. You should obtain a copy for your personal records and understanding.

limited liability company (LLC): A type of legal structure that allows owners the personal liability protection of a corporation and the pass-through taxation and operational flexibility of a partnership or sole proprietorship.

limited partnership: An investment method whereby investors have limits and exercise no control over a company or enterprise; the general partner(s) maintain control and liability.

management: Person who commonly owns or controls the business operations and/or supervises employees.

market: All actual or potential buyers of a product, service, or idea.

marketing: "A social and managerial process by which individuals and groups obtain what they need and want through creating and exchanging products and value with others."[1]

market research: The systematic research, analysis, and reporting of data relevant to a specific element that could impact the organization.

medical records: Documentation needed to provide a chronological record of the client's condition and the appropriateness, effectiveness, and necessity of treatment interventions, and to facilitate a client-centered approach to plan of care.

mission statement: A statement (15 words or less) that describes the why, what, where, who, and how of the organization's goals.

nonprofit: Type of organization that provides charitable services and products for selected individuals or populations with funded or donated monies.

operating core: Persons (employees) who perform the actual hands-on work, such as staff therapists providing therapy services.

operating expenses: The costs involved in operating a business.

operating income: Revenue from operations equal to the volume of sales times the price of what is sold.

organizational chart: The hierarchal and pyramidal graphic representation of the three organizational components. Commonly referred to as a "flow chart."

organizational structure: The organization's outline of ownership, management, operations, and lines of authority.

outsource: To have certain tasks, jobs, etc produced by another company on a contract basis rather than having the work done by one's own company "in-house."

partnership: A legal relationship of two or more individuals to run a company. The two most common partnerships are general and limited liability.

personal selling: A promotional strategy that builds relationships with your customers by personal representation.

place: Where and how you will provide access to your service or product.

policy and procedure manual: An operational tool that acts as a guidebook for practice management.

position: How and where your service or product compares to your competitor's.

price: The cost of the service or product.

product (or service): Any item or features of that item that is offered to the consumer for awareness or purchase.

professional service corporation (PSC): A general corporation that can only be owned and operated by licensed professionals.

profit margin: The amount of money earned after the cost of goods (gross profit margin) or all operating expenses (net profit margin) are deducted; usually expressed in percentage terms.

promotion: The communication of the benefits, price, and place of your service or product.

proprietorship: The most common legal form of business ownership; about 85% of all small businesses are proprietorships. The liability of the owner is unlimited in this form of ownership.

provider network: Organization formed to compete against corporations in acquiring managed care contracts for its members; private practitioners such as occupational and physical therapists. It markets to vendors (third-party payers) for health care service contracts.

public relations: Promotions centered around creating an image about your organization.

purchase expenses (costs): Business items that you paid for and own and that you will deduct or depreciate over time according to the amortization schedule provided by the IRS.

purchases: Documents that demonstrate the amount of a business purchase, such as cancelled checks, credit card summaries, or receipts.

sales and use tax: Tax applied to most sales items.

sales promotions: Marketing promotional incentives that are usually free to the consumer.

self-employment tax: Social security and Medicare tax paid by individuals who work for themselves or in a partnership that acts like the withheld employee taxes by employers.

Service Corps of Retired Executives (SCORE): Retired and working successful business persons who volunteer to render assistance in counseling, training, and guiding small business clients.

small business development center (SBDC): A university-based center of the delivery of joint government, academic, and private sector services for the benefit of small business and the national welfare.

sole proprietorship: A legal entity owned and operated by one person, can have employees and has not filed documents to become a corporation or a limited liability company.

standards of practice: Therapy practice requirements of practitioners for the delivery of occupational or physical therapy services. They can be found through the corresponding national associations, AOTA and APTA.

state sales tax number: Tax identification number assigned by the state board of equalization in order to administer and collect state sales taxes and fees.

strategic partnership: An agreement with another company to undertake business endeavors together or on each other's behalf; can be for financing, sales, marketing, distribution, or other activities.

support services: Persons (employees) who perform supportive work services or tasks for the operating core and/or management, such as the office assistant.

SWOT (strengths, weaknesses, opportunities, threats) analysis: A common evaluative tool utilized in business and health care for determining the viability of a strategy, plan, or idea.

target market: The segment of the market with similar characteristics and needs that is measurable and desirable for an organization to influence.

tax: A percentage of money owed to support the federal, state, and local governments.

tax deferment funds: Investment funds that allow income tax on earnings to be deferred into the future, such as life insurance policies.

tax-exempt funds: Investment funds that earn tax-exempt interest, such as municipal bonds or mutual funds.

tax identification number: Your social security number.

tax qualified products: Investment funds such as retirement plans that allow monies to be invested before paying income taxes on them.

temperament: Personality, attitude, or characteristic traits.

trademark: The name given to any word, phrase, design, symbol, or logo used to market services or products.

unusual occurrence report: A report that is to be filled out by you or your staff any time there is an incident in your clinic. These are confidential documents that are to be used by you and your attorney.

values: Belief systems, ideals, standards, or code of ethics.

variable expenses (costs): Business expenses that are usually controllable and fluctuate with the volume of services and products being utilized.

venture capitalist: Individual or firm who invests money in new enterprises. Typically, this is money invested in the venture capital firm by others, particularly institutional investors.

vision statement: The mental picture of what you and your health care business concept inspires to contribute and achieve.

working capital: The cash available to the company for the on-going operations of the business.

REFERENCES

1. Kotlar P, Armstrong G. *Marketing: An Introduction*. 5th ed. Upper Saddle River, NJ: Prentice Hall; 2000.

INDEX

business receipts, 118-119
business structure, 207
   definition of, 23
   information gathering for, 24
   legal aspects of, 26-23
   organization of, 33-37
   selecting name for, 38-40
   tax status of, 24-26
business success flow chart, 142
buying, business, 73, 75, 174

C corporation, 29
capital, 207
   in business plan, 71
   working, 209
cash basis, definition of, 116, 207
cash flow, 207
   definition of, 116
   improving, 122-123
   managing, 120-122
cash flow projection, 67-68
cash payments, 68
cash reserve, building, 123
Centers for Disease Control and Prevention, human services divisions of, 25
Centers for Medicare and Medicaid Services, 25
certification
   laws and regulations of, 100, 208
   posteducational, 12
certified public accountant (CPA), 120
chamber of commerce, in business name search, 39
checking account, 118
clients, finding, 90
clinical documentation, 97-99
code of ethics, 100, 109, 207
coding, 104, 126-127
Community Mental Health Centers Act, 102
competency, 109
competition, 13
   in business plan, 58-61, 156
   in executive summary, 50
Competition Survey Chart, 59
competitors, identifying, 82
compliance, documentation, 100-101
consultants, 63, 64
consultation, 95-96
consumer needs, 11
contracted services, 140
corporate name, 38-40, 208
corporation, 29-30
   definition of, 207
   organizational chart for, 35
   structure of, 32
costs. *See also* expense(s)
county government databases, 39
cover page, of business plan, 47, 48
CPA (certified public accountant), 120
credit card, 118

DATA Self-Assessment, 3-8
David, Mark, on vision statements, 16
DBA (Doing Business As) name, 27, 38, 208
debt financing, 207
delegation, 123
denial, of reimbursement, 127, 128
desires
   definition of, 207
   in self-assessment, 3, 4, 8
disabilities, laws concerning, 102
discharge summary, 99
documentation, 110
   assessment of, 136

clinical, 97-99
   in evidence-based treatment, 108
   self-assessment, 186-189
   systemic, 100-102
domain name, 38, 207

economic forecasts, 11
educational programs, 11
educational requirements, 12
EIN (employee identification number), 28, 208
electronic resources, 205
   for business concepts, 16
   for business name, 39
   for business plan, 75
   for business structure, 42
   databases, 39
   for getting started in business, 21
   for organizational structures, 37
   search engines for, 39
email postcard, 169
emerging practice areas, 12
employee handbook, 101
employee identification number (EIN), 28, 208
employment tax, 24, 207
entrepreneur
   characteristics of, 2-3
   definition of, 207
entrepreneurial skills, 10
equipment list, 175
equity, 207
ethics, code of, 100, 109, 207
evaluation, in clinical documentation, 98
evidence-based practice, 107-108
Exclusion Authority, 102
executive summary, of business plan, 151-152
exit plan, 208
expense(s)
   in cash flow, 120-121
   definition of, 116, 208
   fixed, 66, 67, 120-121, 208
   indirect, 124
   investing in, 122-123
   operating, 66, 70, 164, 208
   overhead, 124
   purchase, 66, 120, 209
   receipts for, 118-119
   reduction of, 137-143
   tax deductible, 122-123
   variable, 66, 121, 209
expert services, 95-96
explanation of benefits (EOB), 126, 208

facility
   checklist for, 176-177
   design and utilization of, 139
   management of, 102, 106
failure, of new businesses, 12-13
Fair Labor Standards Act (FLSA), 101
False Claims Act, 102
federal employee identification number, 28, 208
federal government, business structure laws of, 25-26
federal income tax withholding, 24
federal trademark databases, 39
Federal Unemployment (FUTA) tax, 24
fee(s), legal, 33
fee schedules, 140
fictitious business name, 27, 38, 208
financial(s)
   in business plan, 47, 63, 65-70, 159
   in executive summary, 50
   reviewing, 135
financial documents, 119

Printed in the United States
by Baker & Taylor Publisher Services

Printed in the United States
by Baker & Taylor Publisher Services